Dear Dr. Roth

Letters to my Website

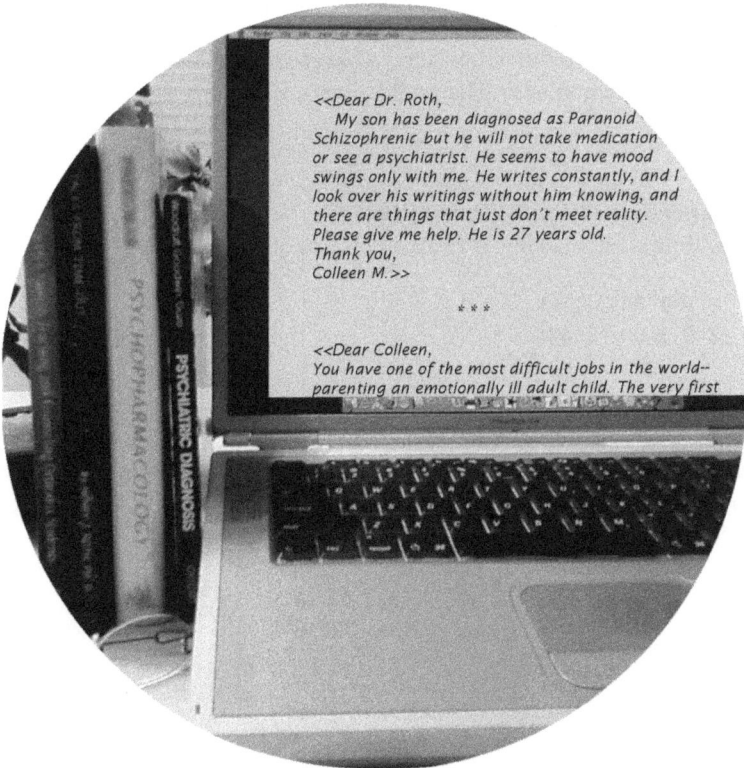

<<Dear Dr. Roth,
   My son has been diagnosed as Paranoid Schizophrenic but he will not take medication or see a psychiatrist. He seems to have mood swings only with me. He writes constantly, and I look over his writings without him knowing, and there are things that just don't meet reality. Please give me help. He is 27 years old.
Thank you,
Colleen M.>>

* * *

<<Dear Colleen,
You have one of the most difficult jobs in the world-- parenting an emotionally ill adult child. The very first

Lorraine S. Roth, M. D.

Foreword by Henry J. Roth, Ph. D.

Roth, Lorraine (nee Lorraine Sharon) 1947-
Dear Dr. Roth, Letters to my Website / Lorraine S. Roth, M. D.

ISBN 10: 0-9785435-1-3
ISBN 13: 978-0-9785435-1-8

1. Psychiatry—Non-Fiction. 2. Psychiatrist—Non-Fiction. 3. Emotional Problems—Non-Fiction. 4. Anxiety—Non-Fiction. 5. Depression—Non-Fiction. 6. Mental Illness—Non-Fiction 7. Schizophrenia—Non-Fiction 8. Phobias—Non-Fiction 9. Panic Attack—Non-Fiction 10. Letters—Non-Fiction. I. Title

10   9   8   7   6   5   4   3   2   1

To Rick

My dear and gracious husband, my sweetheart,
Whose amazing inner strength and intellect
Are matched only by his inexhaustible
Kindness and compassion
Toward everyone he meets.

Will Rogers said,
"I never met a man I didn't like."
Rick never met a man about whom
He couldn't find something nice to say.
I can never stop loving and learning from him.

Introduction

Around the year 2000, I became interested in developing a web page. I included information about my background as a psychiatrist, uploaded my most flattering photograph, and invited readers to ask questions. Over the next several years, hundreds of email letters arrived. Without prescribing medicine or conducting psychotherapy, I gave advice, guidance and information to people who did not know where to turn for the resources to help solve their problems. Much of that advice and information could be helpful to others, so I decided to compile those letters and my responses in this book.

Letters written to newspaper "advice" columns must be edited for length, and are often considerably cut down and streamlined to fit the column allowances. A few of the letters I have included in this book are rather lengthy or "wordy" — but reading the complete letter gives a more accurate sense of the writer's underlying emotions. Therefore, I have left the letters unchanged, including occasional grammatical or spelling errors, except to clarify their message and safeguard confidentiality. Names, geographic locations, and other details such as age, gender, or number of children — anything that might identify the writer — have been changed.

Many of the letters may seem to the reading public to be too bizarre or incredible to be true, but I believe I have eliminated any frankly bogus letters. Sincerity and truthfulness have a certain "ring" to them, which is missing from those written in jest. Every entry herein is from an actual email message that was received on my website. Beyond that, although the reader may feel absolutely certain that some of the letters must surely be fabricated — that no one could legitimately have such a fantastic collection of symptoms — there is nothing in this book that I have not heard, in one combination or another, from my own patients in the thirty years I have been a practicing psychiatrist.

My deepest hope in writing this book is for the reading public to realize how amazingly successful some people can be in spite of towering obstacles of severe mental illness. Individuals who are tormented by mental problems can somehow go through school, receive Masters degrees, supervise large departments of employees, have loving and successful marriages, raise children and take care of their families in spite of recurring symptoms severe enough to require repeated psychiatric hospitalizations. Stories such as those are difficult to believe, but are more common than most people would ever guess; and can serve as beacons of hope for others afflicted with major mental illness, and those who love them.

Finally, I cannot conclude this introduction without addressing the issue of health care. In many of the letters, we see individuals who are working, productive members of society, struggling with severe mental problems, and have no insurance, or their insurance does not adequately cover mental illness. I am hopeful that we will some day soon have a national healthcare program by which everyone is able to procure and afford the basic medical care and medications that they need without non-medical "gatekeepers" deciding what is necessary; and doctors can practice without running up exorbitant costs with excessive testing as insurance against potential malpractice claims.

Thank you for purchasing this book. I hope it provides you with some enjoyable and informative reading, and that you find some value in it.

Very truly yours,
Lorraine S. Roth, M. D.
www.DearDrRoth.net

P. S. Occasionally I referred letter writers to potentially helpful and professionally reliable websites. If any of the links are no longer viable, please accept my apologies.

Foreword

A letter seeking expert advice can be viewed as a first draft from the front lines of a disturbing emotional conflict. In short, such letters represent a conflict-in-motion. By writing a letter to an expert, the individual tries to gain mastery over his personal distress from a position of strength, rather than weakness. Verbal conversations are sometimes difficult to manage because of the intensity of the feelings. For example, a direct question asked of a mental health professional, or even a friend, regarding a particular conflict, may evoke anxious feelings that are threatening for the individual to face. Individuals may become angry, hurt or withdrawn when their conflict touches sensitive feelings.

In contrast to face-to-face verbal conversations, letter-writing is usually perceived in a more objective, non-threatening manner. This is especially the case for individuals who are most comfortable when they are not pressured to speak. Letter-writing can be an important way to externalize emotional conflicts which are too difficult to verbalize. In the process of writing a letter, for the first time, the writer may experience being in control of his conflict as well as his reaction to it. What cannot always be spoken about can be described in a letter in a manner consistent with the writer's personal level of comfort. Many individuals would be reluctant to offer the type of revealing information that can be expressed directly in a letter.

Dr. Roth has collected several dozen letters from the hundreds that were sent to her website. She uses some of the exacting standards of a psychiatric interview and applies them to her responses to the writer's questions. For example, her answers solicit associations between the events in the letters and other factors that may be connected with them. In addition, the answers depend on a variety of factors, including the specific characteristics of the letter, the context of the situation, and understanding the conflict from the writer's point of view. The trick lies in Dr. Roth's ability to provide the letter-writers with something to think about as they begin to develop a more mature understanding of relevant historical and contemporary issues in their lives.

Letters are like classic books — packed with valuable information — if only we could decode their multiple meanings. The decoding value of letter-writing rests in the fact that the individual usually believes he is reporting on a single objective event. He may be unaware that the letter is also subjective; that is, it *reveals* his underlying beliefs and attitudes, as well as *conceals* possible disturbing events that may be too threatening to consciously acknowledge. Samuel Johnson, the eighteenth-century English poet and essayist, pointed out in a letter he wrote in 1777:

> "In a man's letters, you know, Madam, his soul lies naked, his letters are only the mirror of his heart: Whatever passes within him is shown undisguised in its natural process: nothing is inverted, nothing distorted: you see systems in their elements: you discover actions in their motives."

Whether a letter *conceals* important information, and is a few steps removed from a disturbing event, or *reveals* important information, and provides the individual's frame of reference within which he interprets the conflict in the letter, in either case, a letter represents both manifest and latent conflicts, and the individual's attempt to deal with them. Of course it would be impossible for Dr. Roth to address all the issues and embedded themes contained in each letter. However, understanding some of these concealed perceptions can offer the letter-writer an enriching parcel of self-awareness.

The power of this book is that it avoids formulaic responses, and responds to each letter on an individual basis. The letters in this book were written and sent with great expectations. This book memorializes such letters so that their therapeutic value can be recorded. Collectively, these letters represent a casebook of psychiatric issues through the eyes of the letter-writers, and possible strategies through the eyes of a psychiatrist.

Dear Dr. Roth is written for any person interested in understanding and evaluating typical questions that are asked of a practicing psychiatrist about the management of complex problems.

Dr. Roth's thought-provoking answers provide an opportunity for self-discovery and contain themes and patterns that apply to other individuals who face similar challenges. Her straightforward, practical and constructive advice can help to transform a conflict-in-motion into a conflict that is moving in the right direction.

Henry J. Roth, Ph. D.

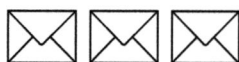

Table of Contents

Part I.

Letters

✉✉✉

Panic Attacks

<< Dear Dr Roth

I was recently diagnosed with having panic attacks. I've been on Xanax for a month now, but it doesn't seem to help at times. What other types of medication are available to treat panic attacks? I've been told that anti-depressants are used. Why are anti-depressants utilized to treat panic attacks; especially when I don't feel I suffer from depression. Patty>>

✉✉✉

Dear Patty,

Depression does not always appear as sadness or moodiness. Depression can show up in different forms, such as anger, chronic pain, anxiety or panic attacks. For that reason, antidepressants can be very helpful in treating panic attacks.

Other classes of medication that can be helpful in treating panic attacks include the anti-anxiety medications, such as the Xanax that was prescribed for you, and even some of the anti-seizure medications.

Best Wishes and thanks for writing.

✉✉✉

<< Dear Dr Roth

Thank You for answering my questions. Again I have another in regard to Panic attacks. I recently started feeling sometimes like butterflies in the pit of my stomach. I feel like it swirls and swirls and the discomfort is always there. I feel like there is something extremely warm in the pit of my stomach right beneath the diaphragm. This feeling goes on for a long time even all day. Like butterflies in my stomach going around in circles and very warm too. I think this is the reason why I lost my appetite because this discomfort won't go away. This started recently. What could be the cause of such a feeling and discomfort? Also, I've noticed that I have a hard time remembering simple things like what I did the day before or what I said a couple of hours ago or what I wrote on my paper. I had to drop one of my college classes because I could not concentrate and could not remember things. What can be causing that? Please help me. Thank You for you're time. Patty>>

⊠⊠⊠

Dear Patty,

It is very important that you get a complete physical exam to determine if there are any problems which are not psychiatric in origin which can be treated. You may need to see a neurologist.

The symptoms you describe—butterflies in the pit of your stomach, loss of memory, inability to concentrate—can be caused by anxiety or depression, but you need to be sure that there is no physical cause which may be treated.

You must be sure and tell your psychiatrist about these symptoms. Xanax and similar anti-anxiety medications have been known to cause memory loss, although that is usually just at the beginning of treatment, or when combined with drinking alcoholic beverages.

If you were experiencing these stomach symptoms before taking Xanax, and physical-medical causes have been ruled-out, then you may need to have a small dose of neuroleptic or anti-psychotic medication added to your regimen. Be sure and discuss this with your psychiatrist.

Best Wishes, and thanks for writing.

Sweaty Palms All Over

<< Dr. Roth I am 25yrs, I am a male who is having anxiety attacks that happen every month or two. This has been happening for about 5 years. I have symptoms that include sweaty palms and all over my body, lack of breath, lack of concentration, stress nervousness, headaches, tightness in chest, and I feel like I am hit by an electric shock in my body. This makes me feel weak at all times. I have done all the tests that were requested such as EKG, EEG, blood work, Citiscan *[CT Scan or CAT Scan]*, chest x-rays, and stress test. these results were all normal so my family doctor suggested to see a psychiatrist that could put me on medication for a period of time.

Wally.>>

⊠⊠⊠

Dear Wally,

All of the symptoms which you listed above can be accounted for by anxiety or panic attacks. However, before that is considered, you may want to schedule a visit with a neurologist—a nerve specialist. It is important to be absolutely certain that a physical problem is not being overlooked.

If you see a specialist such as a neurologist, or at least get a second opinion from an Internal Medicine specialist, and they still give you a clean bill of physical health, then it is time to see a psychiatrist. He may prescribe medication for you, and conduct psychotherapy, which is also very helpful with panic and anxiety disorders.

If it becomes clear that you need psychotherapy, but your psychiatrist does not offer that kind of time-intensive treatment, a

clinical psychologist, psychiatric nurse practitioner, or licensed clinical social worker can be enlisted to help you.
  Best Wishes, and thanks for writing.

✉✉✉

Fighting with Depression

<< Dear Dr. Roth,

I am a 32 yr old female, I am on my 3rd marriage. I have been fighting with depression for most of my life. I stay sad 99% of the time, my husband is wonderful and is trying to understand this but I am afraid to go to a shrink because I know I need to be on meds but I am afraid to go to a shrink because I have (as everyone else has) heard horror stories, but I truly want to get better. Could you recommend anyone in my area?

Thanks
Alicia>>

✉ ✉ ✉

Dear Alicia:

I do not personally know of a psychiatrist in your area, but I am including the answer from the "Frequently Asked Questions" site on my web page, below.

You need not be any more afraid of anti-depressant medication than you are of any other medication. There is no medication on the market, prescription or over-the-counter, which does not have side effects and potentially toxic effects. For example, ordinary aspirin has been known to cause a rare disease, Reyes Syndrome, in a very small number of children when given for flu-like symptoms. Tylenol can cause a fulminating and painful liver inflammation when taken in overdose. Even certain vitamins can become toxic when taken in excessive ("mega") doses.

Anti-depressants are extremely effective, in the 60-80% range, and generally have very tolerable side effects—especially when compared to living with depression. They are also safe when taken in recommended doses. If they were not so safe and so effective when compared to the effects of depression, doctors would have stopped prescribing them long ago.

One of the most rewarding responses a psychiatrist can hear from a patient is, "Now I realize I've been depressed all my life—now that I finally know what it feels like <u>not</u> to be depressed."

Anti-depressants have been lifesavers for literally millions of people who suffer from depression. Psychiatry has over a 50-year history with anti-depressant medication. I hope you will at least go and talk to a psychiatrist before making any decision.

Best Wishes, and thanks for writing.

✉ ✉ ✉

Feel Sad All the Time

<< Hi, Dr. Roth, I think I am suffering from depression. I feel sad all the time. I have lost interest in normal activities. I feel tired all of the time. I have lost interest in my sex life. If you would please just give me advice, I would really appreciate it. Thank you. Loo>>

⊠⊠⊠

Dear Loo,

You may indeed be suffering from clinical depression. It would be very important to be sure that you are not suffering from any physical illness which may be responsible for your depression, such as hypothyroidism (low thyroid hormone) or a pancreatic disorder. There are quite a few medical conditions, and even some medications which can cause depression as a side effect. You should get an appointment for a complete physical check-up.

Once your family doctor has given you a clean bill of health, he can refer you to a psychiatrist who can evaluate your depression more in-depth. Most counties have Health Departments that can offer you services if you do not have a family doctor.

If you are having thoughts of suicide with your depression, you should let your doctor know that you need an immediate appointment, and let him know why.

Best Wishes, and thanks for writing.

⊠⊠⊠

Ending This Thing

<< Hello,

I have a question. I am being treated for depression by my general physician. It seems that no matter what medication they have tried me on, it has no effect on me. I am now at the point that I do not care if I live or not. I have really been think of ending this thing that is called life.

I was talking to a friend about the way that I have been feeling for sometime now and she brought something up that I have been thinking about—she said that it could be manic-depression. My question is how do I know if she is right or not. What would be the signs. I will tell you what I told her.

There are times that I am on top of the world, nothing can stop me, full of energy, have to make myself slow down to be able to even think. But there are times that it takes everything that I have to get out of bed. Some days there are times that I don't see the point in living life, and also just feel like I am worthless, to the point of not eating because of the feeling that I am not worth the food to be wasted on.

But I also have my days that I am just here, can be in a good mood one minute and turn around and be in the world's worst mood for no reason.

Well, I thank you for your time, I hope that I did not confuse you any.

Cammie E. >>

✉✉✉

Dear Cammie,

The symptoms you describe are classic for manic-depressive illness, but that would need to be diagnosed by a mental health professional who could evaluate you in person. Manic-depression is also referred to as Bipolar Affective Disorder, or just Bipolar Disorder. "Bipolar" refers to opposites, such as the North Pole and the South Pole, or the positive and negative charges at each end of a battery. In bipolar disorder, the person's mood or demeanor changes, sometimes rapidly over a few hours, or intermittently at different times of the year. The changes can be very dramatic, unprovoked by any identifiable incident or rational explanation. Bipolar disorder can be characterized by feelings of euphoria, or extreme happiness, then spiral downward into severe depression, often accompanied by suicidal thoughts. Symptoms can also be less extreme — not as euphoric and not as depressed — but still be uncomfortable mood changes that cannot be explained by the situation. Moreover, the elevated and depressed phases do not always appear as happiness or sadness, but may show up as extreme irritability, anger, aggressiveness, hostility, or even violence. Bipolar individuals can become frankly psychotic, with accelerating moods that rocket out of reality and into delusional states, such as feeling that one is a millionaire, and writing checks that can result in serious legal trouble. The depressive phase can have the inability to move out of bed for days on end.

Fortunately, there are many excellent medications that can treat bipolar disorder. You should see a psychiatrist who can prescribe medication if needed. Ask your family physician for a referral, or check with your county mental health agency.

Your thoughts of "ending this thing called life" indicate that that you should seek help as soon as possible. If you find yourself actually thinking of a plan to take your life, or making arrangements for such an event, and no doctor can see you right away, then I recommend going to an emergency room to report your thoughts and mood changes.

Best Wishes, and thanks for writing.

Unable to Fulfill Duties

<<Dear Dr. Roth:

I have a son, he is twenty years old. Since 10th grade in High School he has been unable to fulfill his duties. He said that he was not able to concentrate and that he was very tired. We took him to his primary physician who was unable to improve his condition. Then, we took him to a psychologist who was treating him for a while. My son went also to a psychiatrist. At some point he stopped going. He graduated from High School . He had not applied to any college since he had not decided to study, so we advised him to register in a Community College in order to try to continue studying.

This first semester in the Community College ended and he did not pass any course. He cannot drive, he has refused to learn. He has a girlfriend and friends. Now, he is visiting another psychiatrist, who has prescribed him Buspar and something else. I am really worried and I would like to help him. He is not interested in any activity except for the ones I mentioned before. I find it very weird but maybe I am in ignorance of something.

Thanks a lot,
Worried Mother>>

⊠⊠⊠

Dear Worried Mother:

You said your son is tired and unable to concentrate, since the 10th grade. Was he doing better prior to that time? If there was an acute or sudden change in his personality or energy level and motivation, then he should get a complete medical evaluation. If his personal physician was unable to find any source of his problems, he may need to obtain an evaluation by a neurologist – a specialist in conditions of the nervous system.

Is it possible that he began finding different friends, who may have introduced him to drug or alcohol use? That would be a very important issue to face. If not, he may be having a mood disorder, which can have its onset in the teenage years.

BuSpar is a mild anti-anxiety medication. Your description of your son did not sound as though he is suffering from an anxiety disorder, but there may be symptoms which he has shared with his psychiatrist that you are not aware of. How does your son feel about his psychiatrist? Does he feel he is helping him? If not, he should at least get another opinion.

The best place to get a second opinion and a thorough evaluation is a university medical center, affiliated with a medical school. Those facilities tend to be at the forefront of research and knowledge, both in general medicine and psychiatry. They should be able to diagnose your son's problem and have the latest medications available to treat him, if that is indicated.

But remember – your son is an adult now, and you cannot push him, even if you know he needs help. You do not need to fulfill his every whim or demand; but make sure he knows that you love and support him emotionally.

Best Wishes, and thanks for writing.

⊠⊠⊠

Friend Talks About Suicide

<< I am sending this e-mail concerning a good friend of mine. He has been through a lot in the past year, including his father's death. He is 23 years old and constantly talks about suicide. I feel he needs professional help. He actually agrees, which is good. He doesn't have any health insurance. Is there any way your firm will take payments, or maybe you know of one where he can make payments?

Please contact me... I am desperate. >>

✉✉✉

Dear Desperate,

Depression is normal when one has suffered important losses, and people often work through it without professional help. However, if the depression is leading to thoughts of suicide, it definitely needs to be treated, professionally, and as soon as possible.

There are many myths about suicide—the most dangerous being, "No one who talks about it will actually do it." The majority of suicides were preceded by the person telling someone about it.

If your friend has no health insurance, he should look up the local mental health clinic in your county. Most counties have clinics. He may see a family practitioner first, who can refer him to a psychiatrist or other professional therapist for counseling. Medication can be prescribed which might help the "vegetative" signs of depression — loss of appetite, loss of sleep, loss of concentration, and the most serious, loss of desire to go on living.

Look in the yellow pages under "clinics" or under the white pages for your County Health Department. Also, if there is a hospital affiliated with a medical school in the area, they may be able to treat your friend on a sliding-scale fee basis.

If you can accompany your friend to the initial appointment, to make certain that he goes, and to insure that the suicidal comments are conveyed to the therapist, that would be very helpful. That is important because a person may initially hesitate to describe the true severity of his depression and suicidal thoughts when he is initially interviewed.

If your friend is making active plans for suicide, such as giving away his possessions, writing letters about suicide, or buying a gun, take him to an emergency room for evaluation.

Best wishes and good luck to you and your friend, and thanks for writing.

⊠⊠⊠

Field of Psychology

<< Hello Dr Roth. This is Karen from Springfield, Ca. My concern right now is my daughter, Emmaline. She is 21, in her third year of college, studying to get a B.A. in psychology. The problem is she had not decided what field of psychology she will go into. She does not seem to have a passion for any one field, although she has expressed a concern in helping children. But, she has not decided if school psychology is what she wants to pursue. What suggestions can you give her in deciding a specialty? Are there any internships provided for psychology students? Can she start a job working with a licensed psychologist in private practice to get experience? Any suggestions are welcome. Thank you and good night.>>

⊠⊠⊠

Dear Karen,

Working with a psychologist would be an excellent way for Emmaline to decide what she likes about psychology. She should check with her college guidance counselor to find appropriate resources for such an internship. She may also check with the psychology professors with whom she has studied.

Emmaline is welcome to write to me and ask if she has any more detailed questions about her career. But I would urge her first to contact the many resources which should be available to her at her college.

Psychology usually requires a higher degree of study. Following her Bachelor's degree, a Masters degree and a Doctorate (Ph. D.) may be required to obtain a license to practice as a psychologist in a particular state. Your daughter should be certain about the type of work she would like to do before undertaking a long and expensive course of study.

Best Wishes to you and your daughter, and thanks for writing.

✉✉✉

Crawling Feeling

<< Dear Dr. Lorraine Roth,

I am seeking research that addresses the problem of a crawling feeling under the skin? Included in this most distracting malady is the (sensation) of: Itching, bites/biting, crawling (under the skin). wiggling on back, face, ears, eyebrows, etc., moving all the time. Also, nightmares, can't sleep, scared. This is a very serious affliction that has been dismissed by doctors.

This is for/about my daughter, Keta, age 33, who has been previously treated for anorexia. She believed, at about the age of 12 before the onset of anorexia, that she had contacted fungus under her fingernails and toes (which is questionable). She then self-treated with the harsh treatments to the hands and feet (even left it on all night). I feel that this has affected her neurological system.

Another possible factor is that she was on medication (tegretol) for epileptic seizures during her early elementary school years. Keta feels that life is too difficult to live with this constant crawling under her skin—which she believes to be real parasites. She has told doctors about this and has had it dismissed by them.

It is most important that we find information on this as soon as possible and suggestions on a method of treatment. Is this something about which you are familiar? (Keta is currently in the Milltown, Pennsylvania, area, has a Masters' degree in Business Communications). We need lots of help. Thank you, Dr. Roth.

Frances L.>>

⊠⊠⊠

Dear Frances,

There are psychological conditions which can cause the symptoms you describe. They can be paraesthesias (odd feelings on the skin which are unexplained by physical environment) or tactile hallucinations (feeling something when nothing is there). These can be symptoms of neurological (nerve) disorders or psychiatric disorders.

For example, complex partial seizures (TLE or Temporal Lobe Epilepsy) might cause such symptoms. Withdrawal from alcohol intoxication can include tactile and visual hallucinations (seeing or feeling like bugs are crawling on the skin). Physical conditions such as carpal tunnel syndrome (pressure on the nerves in the wrist) can cause a shooting pain or tingling sensation up the arm. Psychiatric conditions such as schizophrenia, or borderline syndromes can cause transient hallucinations.

Keta may have seen a pediatric neurologist (children's nerve specialist) when she was prescribed with Tegretol. Now she should be evaluated by a neurologist who treats adults. She may need to see a specialist in a large research-oriented academic medical center. It would be ideal if she could be evaluated by a psychiatrist who works in collaboration with a neurologist.

There are probably a dozen or more medications which could bring relief to Keta, including anti-anxiety, anti-psychotic, anti-depressant, and anti-seizure medications. It is not uncommon to require small or moderate doses of several of these medications, and many are quite safe in combination.

Best Wishes, and thanks for writing.

✉✉✉

A Friend with an Eating Disorder

<< dr roth-
i was wondering if you know of any websites with doctors who can help you online. like through e-mail or instant messages. prefferably a doctor who can talk to me about help dealing with a friend with an eating disorder and talk to me about family life and stuff. i would really appreciate it. thanks for your time. i hope to hear from you soon
TapTap>>

✉✉✉

Dear TapTap,

I do not know of any doctors who would take on a regular doctor-patient relationship through e-mail, and I would question the ethical nature of it, particularly if they were charging a fee for the service. If you need to talk to someone at length, check with your local county mental health agency, where you can often find help for a reasonable sliding scale fee. There are also websites which can give you specific information on subjects such as eating disorders.

If you click on the "Health" link of the major websites, they provide some relatively good information in non-medical terminology which you might find helpful. WebMD is a good overall site for general information.

Be cautious of browsing just any web site on the subject of health issues. Some look and sound very professional, but often give inaccurate, or even dangerous, information. Be especially cautious about taking up any "treatments" offered on websites, which can turn out to be unscrupulous scams. In general, the most reliable websites are those from university medical centers, and often have the ".edu" domain suffix. But the best source is a health clinic, speaking directly with a doctor or nurse.

Best Wishes to you and your friend, and thanks for writing.

✉ ✉ ✉

Problems with Therapist

<< Dr. Roth,

As a medical professional, however, not in psychiatry, I am concerned with the therapeutic care of my Significant Other (Being treated for "triggered memories of childhood sexual, emotional and physical abuse"). Currently on prescribed 4 mg/day of Klonopin, 300mg/day of Effexor XR, 2.5 mg of Zyprexa. I have not been pleased with the medications, the way they were prescribed (all begun, except the Zyprexa, at several times the recommended starting dosages), or for the therapy.

And now I have found that the therapist has received a current Censure/Reprimand and her license placed on 2 years probation. The initial charges were more than one count of misconduct, more than one count of malpractice, but the final censure is only for Non-documentation.

My concern from the beginning has caused difficulties because I believe my S.O. feels I am interfering with her therapy. I know the importance of allowing one to control their own therapy, however, I want the best for my loved one. And, lately, she finally seems to be making a bit of progress. But now, I believe my fears are validated. Please forgive me, this sounds like a Dear Abby letter. But now, I am afraid to present this new information, for fear of setting back her progress. I guess I am looking for validation myself, that I am witnessing bad therapy and not overly sensitive myself.

Thank you for your time.

Carren >>

✉✉✉

Dear Carren,

It is most difficult to stand back when we feel that our loved ones are being mistreated, whatever the circumstances. In this case, you know of information that makes you wary of your Significant Other's therapist — and perhaps with good reason. Practitioners get sued for malpractice all the time, but an actual censure is uncommon.

On the other hand, you state, "lately, she finally seems to be making a bit of progress." That is no small accomplishment. It could be very destructive to interfere at this point. You could jeopardize far more than you would help by interfering with a therapeutic alliance which seems to be moving in a positive direction.

There is no telling how it will turn out, but if you see it helping now, and you do not see any evidence that your S.O. is being injured in any way, it would seem to be the wrong time to vent your fears about her therapist. She might resent you to the point that it destroys your own relationship together.

I would advise you to stand in the wings, be supportive and reinforce the positive progress that you recognize. You can always convey the negative information at a later time, but this would seem to be the wrong time.

The combination of medications which your S.O. is taking does not seem to be out of line. She is taking reasonable doses of all meds, and these three different classes (antidepressant, major and minor tranquilizer) are often combined successfully. If she is not having problematic side effects, there is no reason to discontinue them. The meds should be monitored on a regular basis by a psychiatrist who works in concert with her psychotherapist.

Best Wishes, and thanks for writing.

⊠⊠⊠

Money Problem

<<Dear Dr. Roth,

I have a money problem so bad that it caused me my relationship with my future husband. I took out credit cards in his uncle's name to pay the bills and buy food and clothes. When they asked me about it, I lied. I was forgiven for the first time, and then they found out about the second time, and he kicked me out and I need help. How to fix this problem of overspending and doing it by any means. I don't know how to fix my relationship. Help, please! Cindy>>

⊠⊠⊠

Dear Cindy,

You should see a doctor who might be able to help you determine why you overspend. There are some mental disorders in which people spend money in such a way that they get into trouble. This can be a "manic" type of illness, a phase of Bipolar Disorder, for which effective medication is available. You might be suffering from a compulsive disorder, which can respond to psychotherapy along with medication. Or you might be suffering from an antisocial personality which requires a longer-term therapy to develop better ways to cope with stress, observe and appreciate the rights of others, and find a productive path in life.

By all means, seek therapy now before you discover that you can lose more than a relationship. Overspending, and especially taking out credit cards in someone else's name can result in criminal charges. Get help now before that occurs.

Best Wishes, and thanks for writing.

✉ ✉ ✉

Mannerisms

<<Dear Dr Roth.
This is kind of a weird question, but it really bothers my girlfriend. I have always had a very hard time looking people in the eye. I can only glance at them but then glance away. It makes people think I'm hiding something, which I'm not. Any help you can give me would be very nice, and greatly appreciated.
Victor>>

⊠⊠⊠

Dear Victor,

Some mannerisms are hard to break. If everything else in your present situation is okay—your ability to keep a healthy relationship with your girlfriend and other friends, do well in school or on the job, and do the best you can most of the time—then you can feel relatively secure about your mental health.

The mannerism you describe might readily respond to easily accessible treatment strategies. For example, you could take a course in public speaking, or join the Toastmaster's organization, or join another public speaking group. That way you can train yourself to have better eye contact when you speak to people, individually or in front of a group. There are also many different types of psychotherapies, such as Behavior Modification therapy. There are many psychologists who specialize in this type of therapy.

If you suffer from anxiety or depression, or if you have physiological (physical) symptoms such as sweating, palpitations or tremulousness when performing in any way, then you may want to see a psychiatrist who can prescribe medication that can be very helpful. Here is a link that you might find helpful:
Toastmasters International
http://www.toastmasters.org/
Best Wishes, and thanks for writing.

School Project

<<Dear Dr. Roth,

I just wanted to ask you to send me some things on Ritalin. Like what it's about and what does it do to the patients. All the questions I need answered for my school project. Thank you.

Sammy>>

⊠⊠⊠

Dear Sammy,

I cannot do your school project for you, but I am happy to give you some information about Ritalin (methylphenidate). It is widely used by pediatricians and psychiatrists to treat youngsters with ADD (Attention Deficit Disorder) and ADHD (Attention Deficit and Hyperactivity Disorder). It is prescribed for some adult patients who have similar (or residual) symptoms of these childhood disorders.

Best Wishes, and thanks for writing.

⊠⊠⊠

Self-Injury Problem

<<Dear doctor,

I turn to you because I am writing from Latvia and there's not much help I can get here. Psychiatrists here are not very well informed. I have a very big self injury problem I have been dealing with most of my life on and off. It has been on for a long while and no matter what and how hard I try to not do it I still do. The major problems involve:

- biting and touching nails and nailbeds until they bleed;
- scraping my scalp;
- hurting my feet and taking the skin off my feet so I can hardly walk :(
- scratching my legs and not letting the wounds heal, taking the skin off them everytime they try to heal.

As you can imagine, this is interfering with my life in a pretty big way and I was thinking, besides journaling and trying very hard, I could try some medications. What is your experience and what do you suggest? Yes, I do intend to talk to my psychiatrist about medications. Medication is my last resort, I do deal with my problems and issues, I face them and don't try to shove them. I am currently on Paxil 40 mg for my social phobia.

By the way, I am not very sure whether this is impulse-control problem, self-injury or obsessive compulsive. When it comes over me, I cannot stop, I enter a trance-like state and just have to do it, can't resist the temptation even though I know it is harming. It happens on a daily basis. I am not depressed and I cannot understand why I do it since I feel fine. I don't hurt myself because I feel bad about myself or because I feel I deserve to, it's an impulse I cannot control.

I am a 29 year old female.
Thank you for taking the time to read this :)

Janyce>>

⊠⊠⊠

Dear Janyce,

It sounds as though you have a very severe impulse control disorder, or ICD. There are many types of ICD's — pulling out one's hair, which is called trichotillomania; *biting nails is more common; and various kinds of compulsive self-mutilation such as burning or cutting oneself.*

Compulsive disorders are identified by a "build-up" of anxiety that can only be relieved by the injurious behavior. The best way to explain this to people who cannot imagine inflicting pain on themselves is to compare it with a powerful itch that must be scratched; and feeling pain or seeing their own blood somehow provides an immense feeling of relief.

You should definitely get additional help, and possibly additional medication(s) to reduce the tremendous anxiety which leads to the compulsive behavior. Small doses of anti-psychotic medication can be very helpful in cases such as yours, to help alleviate the tension & anxiety. Your doctor can help to adjust the dose with you.

The Paxil you are taking is an antidepressant, and can also be very helpful in reducing your compulsive anxiety, even though you do not feel depressed. Paxil provides adequate relief for some people with compulsive disorders, but it is clearly not doing enough for your severe case.

It is actually very normal not to want to take medication, but sometimes it is necessary. It does not appear that you are adequately medicated at this point. You may also want to get a second opinion from another psychiatrist who can evaluate you in person. That is always a good idea when your symptoms continue to be as severe as you describe. With two psychiatric opinions, you may feel more confident about taking medication, in addition to psychotherapy or behavior modification therapy for impulse control.

Best Wishes, and thanks for writing.

✉✉✉

Essential Tremors

<<Dear Dr. Roth,

I am on a drug Topamax because of what a neurologist calls "essential tremors." What happens is my hands will shake a lot when typing or trying to do some type of movement. I also see a psychiatrist for mental problems. I am not so sure that this isn't mental as well but it does seem to have gone away since I have been on the drug so no complaints.

George>>

⊠⊠⊠

Dear George,

The tremors you describe often run in the family, but they can also be a side effect of a medication you are taking. It is important to discuss all of your symptoms with all physicians who are prescribing your medications. Make sure that your psychiatrist and your neurologist are aware of each other's treatment. Ideally, they should confer with each other about your case.

Topamax, or topiramate, is a medication indicated for treating several different kinds of conditions, including seizure disorders, migraine headaches and excessive sweating (hyperhidrosis). But it is also useful as a second- or third-line treatment for certain kinds of mental disorders such as Bipolar Disorder (extreme mood swings) for patients who cannot take, or don't respond to, first-line medications such as lithium. You did not go into detail about the "mental problems" you are being treated for, but topiramate certainly has the potential to be helping in that area, too.

Best Wishes, and thanks for writing.

✉✉✉

In Love With My Doctor

<< I'm 36,female and have been working with my Dr. (psychiatrist) for 6 or 7 years. In the last year I have fallen deeply in love with this Dr. and while I know that this is not reciprocated I have felt lately that he is not making any attempt to work me through this love. I've broached leaving and seeking therapy other places several times lately but while he never stops me, he assures me that he "knows that I'll stay." I'm feeling very manipulated but also afraid at this time in my life to lose one of the most important people in my life. Then word "love" has never been used and the concept of transference was dismissed in assuring me that what we had was a "real relationship." I have spoken with an aquaintance who is a therapist and also made tentative arrangements to see a recommended therapist. My decision is to stop my appointments with my psychiatrist, 3 days from now, being the day I plan to tell him. But I'm terribly frightened and unsure of how to properly handle this. Please help me.
Pella>>

⊠⊠⊠

Dear Pella,

It is not unusual to feel a strong sense of attachment to one's psychotherapist, because of the frequency of visits and the deeply emotional nature of the problems. The comment which concerned me most was "the concept of transference was dismissed in assuring me that what we had was a 'real relationship'..."

"Transference" is a phenomenon in psychotherapy in which feelings for others from the past are transferred onto a figure in the present. For example, unresolved conflicted feelings that you may have regarding your father, or another prominent figure from your past, are "transferred" onto your psychiatrist. Expressions of transference are expected *to arise during the course of psychotherapy, and identifying the origins of the feeling is an important part of the therapeutic process. If your therapist is allowing you to think that the emotion you are experiencing is "real love," he is misleading you.*

I am relieved to hear that you plan to change therapists. Hopefully your new therapist will help you to work through these emotions, which are normal, but require professional guidance.

You can tell your psychiatrist that you are meeting another therapist to help you work through the feelings you have. You can tell him how much you appreciate all the help he has given you, but it is time for you to assess the progress you have made with him by reviewing it through another professional. I think you are making the right decision.

Best Wishes, and thanks for writing.

✉✉✉

School Project: Abnormal Psychology

<< My name is Lucy Arcadia and I am currently taking Abnormal Psychology in college and we have been assigned a project in which we must pick a topic we are interested in and find professionals in that field and ask them questions. I hope you don't mind answering a couple of questions to help me complete this assignment. It would be greatly appreciated.

Thank you so much for your time.

Lucy Arcadia>>

⊠⊠⊠

Dear Lucy,

You may find the answers to your questions in more detail in my "Frequently Asked Questions" section, under "Psychiatry as a Career." But I shall try to answer them here:

1) Why did you choose to start in the field of Forensic psychiatry?

Forensic psychiatry is a branch of psychiatry that relates to mentally ill (or so they may claim) individuals who have allegedly commited a crime. A psychiatrist attempts to determine the mental state of the accused at the time the crime was committed. That could be a completely different condition from the accused person's present state of mind, at the time the psychiatrist is examining him. Days, months, or even years may have elapsed in the period between the commission of the crime and the psychiatric examination.

2) What do you like most about your profession?

> *The patients! Helping people live more productive lives and feel in control of themselves is beyond rewarding.*

3) Is there any one disorder you encounter that you particularly enjoy studying?

> *Not one in particular. I see patients with a variety of psychiatric disorders and I find satisfaction in working with most all of them.*

4) Can you please give me one shocking or amusing experience you have experienced while working in this field?

> *I had a very disturbed patient who was delusional and hallucinating. Medicine had been only partially successful in helping her. One day, she was involved in a car accident on the hospital grounds, and she suffered a broken arm. As she recuperated from her accident, her psychotic thinking disappeared, and she exhibited normal thought processing. In the years since then, I have occasionally witnessed other instances where sudden severe trauma seemed to have initiated a remission of psychiatric symptoms. One can only speculate on the mechanism for such remission. Perhaps it is a kind of "shock therapy."*
>
> *Good luck in your studies, and thanks for writing.*

⊠⊠⊠

Nightmares

<< Dear Dr. Roth:
My wife and I are middle aged. She has been having nightmares, kicking and hitting in her sleep and thrashing about. I think her problem may be due to her being abused as a child. She has just seen a Psychologist (whom I informed of her past abuse) and he said that he could see no reason for her nightmares. He suggested a sleep disorder test.

Is it possible that her past abuse is *not* causing her nightmares? I would appreciate your answer.

Karl>>

✉✉✉

Dear Karl,

You did not mention whether your wife has had a recent medical checkup. If not, she definitely should. A sleep study may be helpful in determining whether there is any medical problem that can be treated. There are medical problems which can cause sleep disturbance and those should be completely checked out and treated before psychological causes are considered.

If the psychologist you consulted feels that your wife's nightmares are not due to childhood abuse, you should consider getting a second opinion from another psychologist or psychiatrist.

Best Wishes, and thanks for writing.

✉✉✉

Prophylactic Antipsychotic Medication

<< What are your opinions regarding the use of prophylactic antipsychotic and/or antidepressant medications for a patient who has not experienced psychotic symptoms or clinically significant depressive symptomology for over 20 years, but is now being considered for transitional discharge into community outpatient treatment?

Do you know of any resources that would specifically address the issue of prophylactic psychopharmacology?

Gladys>>

✉✉✉

Dear Gladys,

If the patient has truly had no evidence of psychotic or significant depressive symptoms in 20 years, I would not give him prophylactic medication upon his release. Medications are very good, but all have side effects, and there is no reason to give them prophylactically.

If he is coming out into the community for the first time in 20 years, he should have close supervision and observation at least for the first several months, until it is clear that he is comfortably settled in his new environment and has a good support system.

If any signs of relapse are noted, he should be seen by a psychiatrist, and consider starting some medication — or even returning to the hospital for a brief inpatient stabilization. But there is no reason to start medications if he has truly been symptom-free for two decades. Medication is not a substitute for good, appropriate follow-up care.

Best Wishes, and thanks for writing.

⊠⊠⊠

Forensic Evaluation of Ten-year-old

<< Dear Dr. Roth,

I am a Board certified Child and Adolescent psychiatrist working for a State Hospital. I evaluate several children for the court although I am not a Forensic Psychiatrist by training. Recently a request for an evaluation addressing the issue of "Competence" for a 10-year-old with inappropriate sexual behaviors was sent. It was not clear if the Judge wanted to elucidate this youngster's "competence" to stand trial, or how much does this borderline-intelligence boy understand the process. How do you proceed? Do I defer to a forensic psychiatrist?

Dr. Chad >>

⊠⊠⊠

DearDr. Chad,

Forensic psychiatric court cases are fairly uncommon. Because of that, many Officers-of-the-Court (judges and lawyers) recognize the need for a psychiatrist but are unfamiliar with what to expect, and often do not know what to ask.

From your brief description, it would seem that the Court is asking you to determine whether the youngster is competent to stand trial. The definition of competence to stand trial may vary somewhat from state to state—but generally it means that the defendant can understand the charges against him and he is capable of collaborating with an attorney in his own defense. Obviously, these standards would be evaluated differently for a ten-

year-old child than for an adult. A guardian ad litem *may be involved, as well as the child's attorney.*

Although you were only asked to determine "competence," you should find out whether the judge or lawyer also wants your opinion about the child's responsibility for the crime with which he is charged. All of this begs the question of whether the youngster in question actually committed the crime. (You see, it can get very complicated, so you must have a clear idea of what the court wants from you.)

Write to the judge or attorney who sent you the request for an evaluation, and ask for a list of questions which they would like for you to answer. Ask them to be as specific as possible. You should not undertake to do an evaluation nor write a report until you clearly understand what is being asked of you. Once you receive the list of questions, you can determine whether you feel competent to answer them, or whether you should defer to a forensic specialist. If you are not sure where to find someone, you can check out the following links:

American Academy of Psychiatry and the Law
http://www.aapl.org/

American Board of Forensic Psychiatry
http://www.abfp.com/board.html

Best Wishes to you and your client, and thanks for writing.

⊠⊠⊠

Conflicting Feelings About My Doctor

<< Dear Dr Roth,

I am a 29-year-old female who has been in psychiatric treatment for many years. I have Major Recurrent Depression with Borderline Personality Disorder "traits," according to my diagnoses. Presently I am in treatment with a male psychiatrist. The relationship is approximately 1-and-1/2 years old.

I have many conflicting feelings about my Doctor. For the first time in our relationship I am finding myself very upset with him for reasons that I know are inappropriate. As an example, I want him to care more about me than he does. I want him to like me as a person and I don't think he does. I want him to understand how much I need him but he doesn't. He keeps talking about me "getting on with my life" and terminating therapy.

I also have very strong conflicting sexual feelings about him and about sex in general. I don't know if I should tell him the truth about all of these feelings. I am afraid if I do, it will have negative repercussions. Also I am fat and ugly and if I let him know my feelings about him, he may feel repulsed and disgusted even further by me. I have no right having sexual feelings at all. I am fat and ugly. I hate having them and can not stop them. I find myself obssessing about all of these issues. What is your opinion? Thank-you for your time and consideration.

FunyGrl>>

⊠⊠⊠

Dear FunyGrl,

It is not uncommon for patients to have sexual feelings about their therapists after some time. The same holds true for doctors in general. With psychiatrists, it is especially true because of the frequency, intensity, and length of treatment.

It is absolutely unethical for psychiatrists to have sexual relationships, or even personal-friendship-type of relationships, with their patients. It is considered to be taking unfair advantage of a patient who is emotionally or psychologically dependent upon them. The patient is the vulnerable party, and unscrupulous doctors can take advantage of the situation. There is no exception to this ethical code.

You can let your psychiatrist know about your feelings, so that he can help you to work through them. Once it is out in the open, he can help you address these feelings. It is not uncommon for patients—male and female—who have felt dejected and rejected in love relationships to "transfer" these feelings onto their doctor. This is a common occurrence, and is referred to as "transference" in psychoanalysis.

In addressing transference, the patient's feelings for the therapist are analyzed as residual consequences from unmet needs of past relationships. These can include a sense of rejection from cold, emotionally or physically abusive parent-child relationships, or from a lack of satisfying adolescent or adult love relationships.

As for your feelings that you are unattractive, I can only tell you that I have heard the very same self-description of "fat and ugly" from some of the most beautiful women you could ever meet. That is one thing which never fails to amaze me. I have treated young women who are anorectic and have lost fully one-third of their normal body weight, still insisting that they are fat.

During my medical school rotation through the plastic surgery department, I learned never to assume what someone wanted at the first interview. Ask a man with a large nose what brings him to see you, and he may point to a mole on his cheek! People with beautifully formed noses often come in asking for nose jobs. (That is why plastic surgeons frequently require a psychiatric evaluation before conducting any surgery.)

It is a truism that inner sweetness, kindness, and caring for others' feelings is what makes a person beautiful, regardless of their outer appearance. But that also begs the question of whether you are in fact as unattractive as you think. You should share all of these feelings with your psychiatrist. Give him a chance to help you work through them. If you are not satisfied with his response, you may decide to transfer your care to another therapist.

Best Wishes, and thanks for writing.

✉✉✉

Borderline or Something Like That

<< my therapist said i have a personality disorder called Borderline Personality disorder or something like that. i am only 14 and i have no idea what this means. what are the symptoms and what does this mean to me??

NutEBunnE>>

⊠⊠⊠

Dear NutEBunnE,

People with Borderline Personality Disorder (BPD) have a difficult time taking care of things in general and making their relationships work out. They tend to have more trouble dealing with or tolerating friends, teachers, employers, relatives, or romantic partners.

People with this problem tend to be somewhat depressed most of the time, with overall less ability to experience happiness than most people. They may have low-grade anger toward the whole world and toward life in general; their mood can even dip into a major depressive episode, with suicidal thoughts. Under extreme stress, these individuals may have temporary hallucinations, such as hearing voices or feeling paranoid.

People with BPD are vulnerable to substance abuse, to "escape" their depression and anger temporarily. They can engage in other dangerous or self-destructive behaviors, including sexual promiscuity, antisocial behaviors, excessive body piercing, tattooing, or mutilation, such as burning their arms with cigarettes or cutting themselves.

That said, it is important to recognize that your personality is still developing at age 14, and over time with continued support and therapy, it can be molded or guided into a more well-adjusted state. It is good that you are in therapy, as that is very helpful.

Ask your therapist to explain to you how he or she feels that you fit into this diagnosis. Always ask questions! You are entitled to answers. Also, if you are not seeing a psychiatrist who may be able to prescribe medications to relieve your symptoms, along with psychotherapy, you should ask your therapist to refer you to a psychiatrist. There are many medications which are effective for treating depression and the other symptoms of BPD.

Best wishes, and thanks for writing.

✉✉✉

<< well, could you tell me the signs and how it differs from bipolar and skitzos. because my sister is bipolar my dad is something like a manic depressive borderline something. he is just out there and my uncle and great uncle are skitzo. does this make me more at risk. i'm scared. i don't want to be crazy. i know i do things that aren't considered "normal" by most people's starndards of a 15 year old girl but i don't know. i just kinda feel so full but so empty but for some reason i can't open up to my therapist so i don't understand how he could tell any of this by short answers i give like "i don't know">>

✉✉✉

Dear NutEBunnE,

"Bipolar" used to be called Manic-Depressive illness. It refers to mood swings, from very high to very low—beyond the normal range of mood that most people experience. By "skitzo," you are referring to schizophrenia. That is a disorder of thought processes, often including hallucinations, like hearing voices or seeing visions; delusions such as paranoid feelings; and difficulty putting thoughts together and staying on track. Both Bipolar Disorder and Schizophrenia can include hallucinations and delusions, so they are not always easy to differentiate.

There is some tendency for these disorders to be inherited, but that is not always the case. It is not 100% hereditary — even in identical twins it only appears in both twins 60% of the time.

It is important that you discuss your symptoms with a psychiatrist who can prescribe medication, if necessary, that can provide considerable relief to you. Your therapist cannot help you if you do not tell him about all of the symptoms you are having.

If you do not feel you can talk freely to your therapist, you might ask to meet with another therapist. Perhaps a female therapist would make you more comfortable, or just a different therapist. Many of your problems are very treatable, and a significant number of teenagers have feelings similar to yours. Ask your parents or guardian if you can meet with another therapist for a second opinion. Your family doctor may be able to refer you.

Best Wishes, and thanks for writing.

✉✉✉

Unfortunate Predicament: NGRI

<<Dear Dr. L. Roth :

I find myself in an unfortunate predictment that perhaps you can provide an expert opinion on. Right now I am a small fish in a large, unfriendly sea.

During a psychotic state I hijacked a van (I was a marketing executive in a Fortune 500 company) and drove across state lines. Federal charges for kidnapping were brought against me and I spent the next two months in jail. Having no prior criminal history or history of mental illness, my actions came as quite a surprise to friends and family.

I was initially found incompetent to stand trial, then restored to fitness, and found to have been insane at the commission of the crime by an independent (state) psychologist. I would think that the fact I was found incompetent, would make this a very strong NGRI [Not Guilty by Reason of Insanity] case.

My question to you, since you have the background in forensic psychiatry is how many people (percentage) are actually found incompetent? Is that a strong point of my case?

My second question deals with psychopharmacology. If a person was in the throes of a severe depression (which I began suffering from about 6 months before the crime was committed — was even hospitalized for suicidal ideation) and placed on an anti-depressant without a mood stabilizer... could they experience an induced mania. I believe the American Psychiatry Association described a similar phenomenon as BiPolar III. What is your professional opinion?

If it is of interest, I will add that I took the medications sporadically as well because I was convinced I was the epicenter of evil and that the devil controlled me. I was placed on Celexa and then Paxil. Truthfully, we moved to Seattle because of an opportunity for a promotion in my company, and do not have a strong network in place. I did not even call my wife after I was arrested because I believed I deserved to be there. She had approximately 3 hours to find an attorney for my bond hearing (the same attorney we have subsequently and unfortunately been stuck with due to financial constraints).

My wife and I have been married for nine years — talk about a strain on the marriage! I have suffered in the Federal Prison system under unimaginable conditions because of a crime I never would have committed had I been well. There is absolutely no motive that I can conceive of. Is it really fair that I'm branded for the rest of my life with a felony because of an illness I had no control over?

I look forward to your response. I have resorted to doing most research on my own. My attorney is out of his league. I am also interested in information on your fees for testifying should we work out a mutual relationship. Thank you so very much in advance for your consideration and response to this matter. Life as I know it truly is on the line for me.

Sleepless in Seattle,

P.S. The charges are in California>>

⊠⊠⊠

Dear Sleepless,

You have certainly done your homework well. Most of the points you make are quite valid, except for the following: A finding of incompetency (not competent to stand trial) is not the same as NGRI. One could be found Not Guilty by Reason of Insanity, yet perfectly competent to stand trial. Competence is judged at the time the trial rolls around, and depends on the defendant's ability to understand the charges and collaborate rationally with his attorney.

On the other hand, a defendant who was "sane" at the time of the crime could have a recurrence (or new onset) of mental illness after the fact, and by the time the trial took place might not be competent to stand trial.

Regarding your first question, there is a very, very small percentage of successful NGRI cases — perhaps one percent. However, that is probably because lawyers attempt to invoke the insanity defense when they have no other defense to use. For example, a man who killed someone in a fit of rage is unlikely to find a sympathetic jury, even though a psychiatrist may insist he was severely depressed at the time of the crime.

Your case, in contrast, sounds like a classic NGRI case, from the small amount of information contained in your letter, although I have not examined you. I say that because the crime sounds bizarre, with no apparent motivation that makes any rational sense; and assuming the lack of a history of criminal behavior in your past.

That brings us to your second question about psychopharmacology. Anti-depressant medication is well known to have the ability to "trigger" a manic episode in persons who are predisposed to mania. Often there is no warning. That is why a psychiatrist who first prescribes an anti-depressant to a patient should always follow up frequently during the first few weeks of therapy.

According to your letter, some months before the crime, you experienced an episode of severe suicidal depression requiring hospitalization; then had paranoid thoughts about the devil and the epicenter of evil; then you were placed on Celexa and Paxil. Both of those medications are anti-depressants, and would not be expected to treat psychotic or paranoid thoughts. Either or both of those medications, which are very effective antidepressants, are capable of triggering a manic psychosis in a predisposed individual.

You must find a qualified forensic psychiatrist licensed to practice in your state who can examine you in person and put all of the information together into a report for the Court. If your lawyer cannot help you, you may check the following link:

American Academy of Psychiatry and the Law
http://www.aapl.org/

Best of luck to you and thanks for writing.

⊠⊠⊠

(One-Year Later: Follow-Up to Unfortunate Predicament)

Dear Sleepless,

I was reviewing some of the letters I have received over the past year or so, and ran across yours again. I was wondering how you are doing? I hope all went well for you in your difficult situation.

⊠⊠⊠

<< Dr. Roth:

Very thoughtful of you to follow-up! Unfortunately, the legal system is not as understanding of mental illnesses as I would have hoped. Considering the climate of the times as well as the Andrea Yates[1] case, I decided not to gamble that I would win an insanity defense. I love my wife and my family way too much to risk being separated from them possibly for years. I took a plea bargain that includes no jail time, but 30 days of home detention and 5 years supervised probation. I guess that Hinkley[2] really messed it up for anyone else hoping to get off on the insanity plea (those legitimately needing it)...I guess all I can do is work toward positive change regarding the legal system. My eyes have been opened! Again, thank you for your concern. Best of luck to you personally and in your professional endeavors (I have no doubt you are sucessful at what you do!).

Take Care,
Marty in Seattle

✉✉✉

---

[1] Andrea Yates drowned her five young children on June 20, 2001, in their family bathtub. Initially convicted of first degree murder in 2002 and sentenced to life in prison with parole possible after forty years, her conviction was later overturned on appeal. On July 26, 2006, a Texas jury ruled Yates to be not guilty by reason of insanity [NGRI], and consequently committed to a high-security mental health facility.

[2] John Hinkley attempted to assassinate President Ronald Reagan on March 31, 1981. He was found innocent by reason of insanity and was committed to St. Elizabeth's psychiatric hospital in Washington, D. C.

Dear Marty,

I am both sad and relieved for you at the same time. You probably saved yourself and your family a great deal of heartache and expense by choosing the path you did. I applaud your courage.

Good luck to you, and best wishes to you and your family.

✉✉✉

Felonies Ruin My Chances?

<< Dear Dr. Roth

I am a third year college student, and would like to become a psychiatrist, however I am faced with a question. You see before I finished high school I got into trouble with the law on two occasions — both were felonies. I am now 32 years old and for the last several years have done well to get my act back together. I am doing very well in college. My question is, does those 2 felonies totally ruin my chances to become a psychiatrist. I really need the answer, and would like to hear back from you soon.

Sincerely george!!>>

⊠ ⊠ ⊠

Dear George,

I would guess that your chances of getting into medical school would depend on the nature of the felonies and the standards for training and licensing physicians in your state. Those may be different from state to state. You will have to explore these criteria in the different states in which you would like to obtain a license to practice.

Once you are accepted into a medical school, with your past record out in the open, you may be able to get into a residency training program in psychiatry, or other specialty. However, once again, you would have to check with the different programs in each institution. For example, you may be accepted for a residency in psychiatry in one program, but not in another.

Here are two links which you may find helpful in your quest:

American Medical Student Association
http://www.amsa.org/

Association of American Medical Colleges
http://www.aamc.org/

Good luck to you in the future, and keep up the good work.

✉✉✉

Should I Still Be On It?

<< Hi Dr.

The problem I am facing is that I have been on pretty much ALL of the anti-depressant drugs and have been on 40mg. of Prozac for approx. 5 years. I have been reading and am wondering if I should still be on it for this long? I have been having MANY side effects, especially lately. I feel that I should probably be weaned off this drug but do not want to go through the withdrawal symptoms without Dr. supervision. I am located in Prairie Hill (approx. 60 miles north of Springfield). I NEED to see somebody who has experiences in taking somebody OFF of these types of drugs and treating with alternative methods. Any help would be greatly appreciated.

Thanks,

Belinda >>

⊠⊠⊠

Dear Belinda,

You are wise to avoid withdrawing from medication without a doctor's supervision. Who is prescribing the Prozac for you now? If you are getting it from your family physician, ask him if he can refer you to a psychiatrist for a review. He can design a safe withdrawal schedule while observing for any relapse in the symptoms for which the antidepressants were initially prescribed.

There are many new antidepressants coming out on the market year after year. If you continue to require medication, it is possible that there is an antidepressant that you have not taken that might work better for you, with less side effects, than the Prozac. Prozac is an excellent antidepressant, and many people take it without difficulty. However, if you are experiencing side effects which you find unacceptable, then it is time for a change, or at least a trial of another medication.

There are several family physician's groups in your area that you can contact for more information, if you are not seeing a personal physician. They should be able to refer you to a psychiatrist. You can also check the white pages for your county mental health clinic.

Best Wishes, and thanks for writing.

✉✉✉

Obsessing Over Grades

<< Hi, my name is Nicole French. I am a student at a Technical School and I need your help and advice in solving something I did. I need your help or advice because I kind of feel bad or good for what I did. I am very confused and need your help because I keep thinking about this everyday and every minute. The problem is that I got a "B" for English class in school, but I feel that in a way I deserve this grade and in a way, I do not deserve this grade. I feel this way because I am trying not to cheat in school because I used to do this in high school and regret doing this. I am trying to change. The problem is that for the test even though they were open book and open notes test, the professor would put 6-8 questions on 2-3 tests that did not have the answers to them from the book or notes. So because of this, I would check my ungraded test with another classmate's graded test. By the way, the last test was the easiest test. I did not check my test with the other classmate's test, because the last test had all the answers in the book and he did not make any right answers wrong. I got an 88% for the last test, which is a B. Along with the test, if we do all the homework than he will raise our overall grade to a letter grade higher because in his class the tests make up 67% of our final grade and the homework will make up 33 % of our final grade. I did all of my homework as well.

Dr. Roth, if all three of his tests were not like that and they were like the last test, then I would have not checked my test with another classmate's test. Do you think that I was cheating on the test or not? Do you think that I did deserve this "B" for the class or not? I was scared to turn in my test like that also because we only have 4 tests and it is like if I got a D or an F for one test, then I would have probably done bad in this class. But, I do not think that this was my fault. It was the prof. fault, it is not fair to put test questions that are not in the book or in the notes. Please respond to this e-mail. Thank you so much. Have a nice day and please take care.>>

⊠⊠⊠

Dear Nicole,

I think that you are worrying too much about this test, grade, and professor. It is good that you have a good conscience and do not want to cheat; at the same time, the professor's seeming unfairness makes you feel that you need to make up for it.

College classes as well as life itself are like that. When you go out in the world and get a job, you may feel the same way about paying income taxes — lots of people do. They work hard and consider themselves honest, but ask why they should tell the government everything they make and give it away? They feel justified in holding back because they may disagree with the government spending. In any case, the honest thing to do is to do what is required of you.

You may want to consider talking with your professor. Ask him about any questions which you feel were graded incorrectly, or which were not covered in his lectures nor in the textbook. If you approach him in a mature, calm manner, and ask how you can get some help, he should be very happy to help out.

If I tell you not to worry too much about this one grade, and you continue to worry and obsess over it, then you may need to talk to a professional in your area. Is there a health clinic affiliated with your school, or a mental health clinic run by your county where you can see someone on a sliding scale? You may find that to be very helpful, if you cannot afford to see a private therapist.

Best Wishes, and thanks for writing.

⊠⊠⊠

<< Hi, this is Nicole French again. Where can I find free on-line therapist and counselors to help me with my problems because I do not have money and is still worrying a lot over the situation about me with the math and english classes. I really need a lot of help because I still keep worrying about this everyday. However, I do not have no money at all to pay for an on-line therapist or counselor. Thank you so much! Have a nice day>>

⊠⊠⊠

Dear Nicole,

Your school should have counselors available for you to speak with. You should have an advisor assigned to help you, and he or she should be able to recommend a counselor. Your school may also have a student health clinic where you can find a mental health counselor or therapist.

If you do not wish to go to your own school counselor, go to a local county mental health agency, which you can find in the yellow pages under "clinics" or "mental health" , or in the white pages under your County name. They may be able to provide you with a counselor at a nominal fee, or on a sliding scale fee, or possibly just a small co-payment.

Best Wishes, and thanks for writing.

⊠⊠⊠

<<Hi, this is Nicole French. I did find many mental health services and mental health counslors in the real yellow pages of Alta Vista County. If I get a mental health counselor, what types of things will this person be able to provide for me? Will they be able to tell me if I was cheating or not?>>

⊠⊠⊠

Dear Nicole,

A mental health counselor should be able to help you deal with your feelings and your own value judgments about yourself — whether they are too harsh or even accurate. They can help you work through these anxieties and feel better about yourself and your school work. In time, those feelings will extend to all of your endeavors, and will enable you to enjoy more success and satisfaction in whatever you undertake to accomplish.

Best Wishes, and thanks for writing.

⊠⊠⊠

Research Paper: Bipolar Disorder

<<Hi Dr. Roth,
I am currently attending nursing school at a state University. I am currently working on a research paper on Bipolar disorder. For my research project I am required to conduct several short interviews with someone who is qualified in the area. I'm not sure if you're familiar with Bipolar disorder at all, but I came across your website and since you specialize in Psychiatry, I am interested if you would be able to possibly answer a few questions by e-mail. I know that you are busy and I would greatly appreciate any help that you may be able to offer. Thank you for your time,
Candace>>

⋈⋈⋈

Dear Candace,

I would be happy to answer a few questions on the subject of Bipolar Disorder. First, however, let me refer you back to my website to look over the "Frequently Asked Questions" section. You may find a lot of information there.
Best Wishes, and thanks for writing.

⋈⋈⋈

[Candace must have found all of the information she needed in the FAQ section, because she did not write back!]

Real Psychiatric Education?

<< Hi Dr.Roth

Can you tell me if an ABPN certification is a real psychiatric education?

Is this a weekend test and certification company?

Thanks

N. P. Sheffield >>

⊠⊠⊠

Dear N.P.,

ABPN certification is awarded to Diplomates of the American Board of Psychiatry and Neurology. Testing and certification follow an accredited psychiatric residency training program which generally runs for four years following medical school, and includes training in Internal Medicine and Neurology.

Following graduation from an accredited medical school, a Medical Doctor (M. D.) can apply for a psychiatry (or other specialty) residency training program. That may be appended by another year or more of fellowship training.

Best Wishes, and thanks for writing.

⊠⊠⊠

What Forensic Adds

<< Dear Dr. Roth;

I am an attorney in New York City. I am trying to find out what forensic adds to psychiatry. I have read the definition on your website:

> **Forensic psychiatry** *involves the determination of sanity during the commission of a crime; mental competence to stand trial; competence to write a will (also known as testamentary capacity), and competence to gain custody of children. There are other areas of mental functioning or capacity which may require evaluation by a forensic psychiatrist.*

What does that have to do with treating people's medical problems?

Thank you
M. G., Attorney-at-Law>>

⊠⊠⊠

Dear M. G.,

"Forensic" refers to "legal" or "public" argument or debate. It does not "add" anything to psychiatry—but the opposite is true: Psychiatry adds understanding to forensic issues.

There are precedents going back to Biblical times which suggest that it is inhumane to punish someone who, simply speaking, did not understand the "wrongfulness" of his actions; or, if he did understand it, may not have had the capacity to control his actions. Psychiatry helps to shed light on a person's mental functioning, capacities or abilities.

It is clear when you are dealing with a very young child, a toddler, for example, who takes another child's toy and refuses to give it back. No one claims that the toddler should understand the law relative to possessions and ownership. That determination is infinitely more difficult when an adolescent fatally shoots another child. The gravity of the incident begs for more thoughtful examination.

When one is dealing with adults who have a history of mental illness, it is not always clear whether they should be held responsible for an illegal act or not. A psychiatrist who has treated patients with schizophrenia, mania, and other mental illnesses can help to sort it out for the courts. People who are unfamiliar or uncomfortable around mentally ill patients may find them to be an object for derision, scepticism, or amusement. A forensic psychiatrist can help to shed light on the patient's condition and how it related to the alleged crime, so that the attorney, judge and jury can better understand and come to a reasonable conclusion.

With respect to your last question, it is sometimes possible to help an accused person, medically. The defense lawyer may ask the judge to commit the patient to a hospital or clinic where they can be treated while awaiting trial. Medication can help to stabilize a psychotic patient, who may then be competent to collaborate with his lawyer and aid in his defense.

I hope this has been helpful. Please do not hesitate to write back if I have not adequately answered your concerns.

Best Wishes, and thanks for writing.

✉✉✉

Prozac vs. Paxil

<<Doctor: I had a very bad panic episode which converted to depression three years ago. I took 10mg Paxil which got rid of the panic and depression but I didn't like the side effects and stopped taking Paxil after seven weeks.

A few months ago my I started to experience severe anxiety and depression again. My main problems were: anxiety, obsessive feelings of guilt and worry and some melancholy. I started taking 10mg Prozac three weeks ago and also take 10mg Serax to help me sleep a couple of nights a week.

I chose Prozac because after reading many articles about it, I felt it had fewer side effects than other SSRIs [Selective Serotonin Reuptake Inhibitors] and I would be more likely to continue taking it for six to eight months. I have had a few side effects from Prozac but I also don't feel it is working as well for me as the Paxil did.

My question: Is Prozac appropriate for people like me whose primary symptom is severe anxiety? Thanks. Rita.>>

✉✉✉

Dear Rita,

Prozac and Paxil are very similar. The side effect "profiles" are determined from the reports by thousands of patients and their doctors, and do not occur in everyone who takes them. In other words, if an average weight loss occurs in 15% of people who take

Prozac, that does not mean you will lose weight—some patients even gain weight.

The most important criterion in determining the right medication for you is how it works for you. *If the Paxil worked better than the Prozac, by all means, take the Paxil. If the side effects are intolerable, try a different antidepressant. If the side effects are tolerable enough to take it for a few weeks, you might take it for a few weeks to get rid of the anxiety and depression, and then switch to Prozac, or another antidepressant that has more tolerable side effects.*

Are you working with a psychiatrist who is prescribing these medications for you? You did not mention that. If you are obtaining these on your own somehow, please contact a psychiatrist who works with psychiatric medications (as opposed to a psychiatrist who limits his practice to psychoanalysis or "talk therapy").

The first place to look if you do not know where to find a psychiatrist is to ask your local family doctor for a referral. If you do not have one, look in the white pages under your County health clinic or mental health clinic. If there is a hospital near you which is affiliated with a medical school, that is an excellent place to get help.

Best Wishes, and thanks for writing.

✉︎✉︎✉︎

Considering a Career in Psychiatry

<< Dear Dr. Roth,

I am a transitional-year medical resident at a private clinic hospital who is considering a career in psychiatry. I was close to applying for residency in psychiatry last year but backed off secondary to worries about the trends in the field away from psychotherapy and toward brief medication management visits. I received my undergraduate degree in literature and philosophy, have a strong interest in these fields and in psychology, and feel extremely interested in the inpatient psychiatry patients and in how their minds work. I loved my med school inpatient rotations but it seemed like the attendings were maybe too busy to ever talk to the patients outside of the narrowly focused psychiatric examination for H&P [History and Physical] and daily notes. If you could give me some feedback on how you feel about the field and in particular on how you or your colleagues involved in inpatient psychiatry feel about these issues, I would very much appreciate it.
Thanks,

Sharon>>

⊠⊠⊠

Dear Sharon,

My colleagues may feel differently, so I cannot speak for them. Personally I feel it is a mistake to worry about "trends" in psychiatry. You have too many options open to you. If you take an academic position with an eclectic institution—one that teaches an overview of all types of psychiatric practice and therapies—you can practice in the manner that you feel most comfortable. If you take a position with a large government insitution, such as a state hospital or veteran's hospital, you will likely have a larger caseload. However, there is ample opportunity to share coverage with other doctors and to make time for a number of psychotherapy patients with whom you choose to work.

Private practice is still a good option. Don't let anyone tell you it is difficult in a managed-care environment. Private practice is extremely rewarding, but you must be patient. It takes time to build a thriving private practice. Choose an area of sound economic base, and avoid taking patients who cannot really afford to pay, even if they are willing to go into debt, such as credit card debt, to pay you. You will not be doing them any favor—you will make their problems worse. Have a wide referral base so that you can steer such patients toward clinics that offer a sliding scale. You may even want to donate a portion of your time for some sliding scale patients as part of your own contribution to the community.

Above all, I recommend that you avoid any contract which you may be tempted to sign with an HMO (Health Maintenance Organication). I personally believe that the concept itself is unethical and promotes poor medical care. Most of these organizations are run as businesses, and make money by charging the highest premium possible while giving the least amount of care. You can build a very successful practice without helping non-medical profiteers amass a personal fortune at your patients' expense.

I would like to say one more thing about psychiatry, and about Medicine in general: There is no more secure or rewarding profession anywhere in the world. Medical doctors educated and trained in properly accredited institutions are welcome everywhere. Psychiatry is a specialty that is in great need, with vacancies abounding. Few enough medical graduates are interested in psychiatry, so if you are, I hope you will pursue it. You will never want for material or spiritual security if you practice any field and any specialty of medicine. Patient care, teaching, or research provide diversity and are all available to you.

    Best Wishes, and thanks for writing.

✉✉✉

Husband Viewing Internet Porn

<< Dr. Roth,

I don't even know if you can answer my question, but I'll ask anyway. I am 35 years old, mother of 2 darling twin girls. This is my second marriage — the first was emotionally abusive and included infidelity. My present husband is not like that, he's sweet, caring, loving, supportive, etc. I suffer from very low self esteem and a lot of trust issues with men (my father was abusive also — if that matters). I also suffer with anxiety and constant worry, always in the stress mode. I tried Prozac for awhile, but it didn't seem to help.

Anyway, lately I've felt very anxious about my husband viewing pornographic material on the internet — I found this out recently. I confronted him and told him it bothers me, and he says I'm making a big deal out of nothing. I know men are visually stimulated, and intellectually I can understand his interest in looking at naked women every chance he gets — on tv, magazines, the 'net, whatever.

Why does this bother me so much? It really makes me crazy! I feel like he's committing emotional adultery. It makes me feel ugly, because my body isn't as nice as these other women. I'm tired of feeling this way, but I don't know how to find a good psychiatrist or psychologist in my area, or if my insurance would cover it. Margie>>

⊠⊠⊠

Dear Margie,

Let me first address your comment about your father: Yes, it does matter. When someone is brought up under constant criticism, severe verbal, physical or sexual abuse, their view of life is depressing from the very start. It often stays that way into adulthood. Your mood may be somewhat depressed even when things are going well; and a chronic, low-grade depression may actually feel "normal" to you.

It is possible that there were "clues" that your present husband enjoyed looking at porn before you married him, and you may have unconsciously "suppressed" those clues. There is a psychological phenomenon known as "repetition compulsion" in which case someone repeatedly gets into the same unpleasant situation over and over again, unconsciously hoping for a different ending – a "happy ending" – at last. For example, a woman whose father was an alcoholic may marry an alcoholic, divorce him, and remarry yet another alcoholic, again ignoring the "red flags" that everyone else can see in advance.

If your present husband is as good of a helpmate as you describe, you must keep that in the forefront of your mind. If he is faithful and loving, and you find him satisfying in the most important ways to you, then try to keep your feelings in perspective. It is quite common for someone to have felt excited or sexually attracted to an actor or actress in the movies, or on television, or even an acquaintence that they know. That is human nature, and that alone should not destroy an otherwise rewarding marriage.

Let me also address your symptoms of anxiety and depression. It is possible that you did not try an adequate dose of Prozac, or you did not stay on it for long enough. Ask your family physician for a referral to a psychiatrist, because there are many more antidepressants on the market that could provide you with significant relief from your low mood and anxiety. Your feelings of low self esteem could lift if your depression were successfully treated — they often go hand-in-hand.

If your insurance does not cover a psychiatrist, check in your area for a county mental health clinic. They should have a sliding scale fee that you can manage. The ideal solution would be for both you and your husband to see a counselor together. You might broach the subject by saying you are not trying to change him, but by attending together, you can learn how to deal with his peccadillos, and he with yours.

Best Wishes, and thanks for writing.

✉✉✉

I Want to be a Child Psychiatrist

<< I want to be a child psychiatrist. Should I choose pre-med, or psychology as my major? I'd really appreciate it if you could help me.

Thank you for your time,
Yolanda >>

⊠⊠⊠

Dear Yolanda,

Check out the "Frequently Asked Questions" section on my website regarding psychiatry as a career. I think most of your questions will be answered there. If not, feel free to write back and ask additional questions.

Good luck in your career, and thanks for writing,

⊠⊠⊠

Help Out a Struggling Writer

<< Dr. Roth

I'm not sure if you'd be willing to answer this question, you may well think I am strange. I am writing a book in which a person is given a drug that disables the body but leaves the mind coherent. I haven't found any useful information on the matter. Most likely because I have no clue exactly what I am looking for. Would you be interested in helping out a struggling writer? Any info on an applicable drug and perhaps a brief description of it's effects would be greatly appreciated, and I will be sure to mention you as an information source. Thank you in advance.

Lin

Bangor, Maine >>

⊠⊠⊠

Dear Lin,

A better source for the information you seek can be found at the following website:

American Board of Forensic Toxicology
http://www.abft.org/

Good luck in your career, and thanks for writing.

⊠⊠⊠

Researching Careers

<< Dear Dr. Roth:

Please send back with questions answered. This will not be published, nor will your name or any other personal information be disclosed. This is for my personal use only. The aim of these questions is to provide myself with information about the psychiatric careers. I am a high school student researching careers for personal reference. Please respond as soon as possible. I apologize for any inconvenience this may cause you. Thank you for your time. Lily >>

1. How long have you been working in this field?

   Since 1979 as a medical doctor, and as a psychiatrist since 1983.

2. Where did you get your education and how long did it take?

   Check out my website — it's all there!

3. What are your major job responsibilities?

   Evaluating and treating psychiatric inpatients and outpatients, sometimes treating their other medical problems as well. And filling out lots and lots of forms!

4. How does your job compare to other jobs in the health field? Consider your salary benefits, and opportunities.

There is no comparison to any other job in the world, if you are interested in medicine and have a strong aptitude for science and math, and good "people" skills.

5. What are the fringe benefits of your job?

Check out my website — it's all there!

6. How did you select this occupation?

I didn't select medicine — it selected me. I was going to major in Nursing, then Biology, with plans to teach — but my college professors encouraged me to go into Medicine. I never thought I was up to that; but they did. (Thank you, Dr. Avin Brownlee and Dr. Joyce Fan.)

7. What are the opportunitites for advancement?

You can "advance" administratively, if you are interested in that. For example, you can pursue a position as a department head or hospital official, or direct a research program or institute of higher learning.

8. What are the hours? Do you have any control over your work schedule?

You make your own schedule as a private practitioner. You may ask others to follow your patients while you are on vacation, and you do the same for them. Working for an institution, such as a state hospital, you arrange your schedule with them, usually part-time or full time.

9. Is there job security?

There is 100% job security as a physician, in the sense that you are welcome anywhere in the world. You will never want for work. However, if you are working as a salaried employee of a state or federal institution, they may cut back or "downsize" if their funding is cut, just as any business might. But psychiatrists, especially, are in short supply all over the country.

10. Are you satisfied with the salary you receive?

Yes.

11. Is the job structured, or is there flexibility?

Most all physician's jobs are flexible to a certain extent. Full-time vs. part-time, private practice vs. government or academic positions — there is a great deal of flexibility.

12. Do you feel that you are respected in your position?

Yes. Actually, people love to make fun of psychiatrists, but that has never affected my sense of being respected. We like to make jokes about other doctors, too (but especially about lawyers).

13. What do you like and dislike most about your job?

Love the patients, hate the paperwork!

14. What are your future goals?

I have accomplished all of my goals. My future goal is to continue what I am doing as long as I am able.

15. What do you like to do in your free time?

I greatly enjoy spending time with my family. I also love to read books — fiction and historical; and write.

16. What would you say are your most important accomplishments to date?

Raising my three children; quitting smoking.

17. If you had the chance to make a change in your career, what would you do and why?

Nothing different regarding my career at all. I am very satisfied. I would try to have made more time to spend with my family, but psychiatry is pretty good in that respect.

I hope I have answered your questions satisfactorily, but if not, feel free to write back again.

Good luck on your Vocational Research Assignment, and thanks for writing.

✉✉✉

More Questions About Psychiatry

<<My name is Jared if you can possibly reply to these questions i have on the topic of psychiatry then i would very much appreciate it, thank you for your time.

Jared.>>

1. What type of preparation (if any) did u have to go through to be in this profession?

Check out my website — it's all there!

2. What type of post-high school education was required?

Ditto #1

3. Was it necessary for you to do be an intern with someone in this profession or in a profession similar to it?

Ditto #2

4. What type of special skills does it take to be in this career?

Patience, good "people" skills, and an aptitude for science and math.

5. What are some responsibilities associated in your career?

You are responsible for the results of your medical treatment and advice. You have a responsibility to keep up with the latest information in your field. You have a responsibility to be honest with your patients and their families. You are responsible for maintaining a professional relationship with your patients and their family members.

6. What are some challenges you face everyday in your career or have faced in the past?

The primary challenge in medicine is to make an accurate diagnosis when the signs and symptoms do not fit exactly with the textbook description of the illness. The next challenge is to choose the right medication and dose so that the patient gets better with a minimum or no side effects to cause more problems.

7. When did you feel you wanted to pursue a career as a psychiatrist?

Interesting question. I originally wanted to go into nursing or biology. Once in medical school, though, I wanted to be a plastic surgeon — it appealed to my artistic nature (in my childhood I wanted to be an artist). But I did not think I could personally do a good job raising a family along with the punishing schedule of training required for surgery. It was not until I actually began a rotation through psychiatry that I realized how "right" it was for me. I loved the idea of saving a person's mind, and was amazed at the array of medication that could do that. Also, the schedule of training in psychiatry tended to be more relaxed and more conducive to raising a family.

8. Did you have any reservations about it?

None whatsoever. I have never regretted my decision to go into psychiatry.

9. And Last...If I were to take an interest in this career and pursue it as a job what are classes that I could take in high school to further my chance of success in this career?

Take all the science and math courses that you can in high school.

Good luck in your studies, and thanks for writing.

✉✉✉

Sexual Harassment

<< How should a smaller, less athletic-type subordinate retail salesperson work/bond with a large athletic power-hungry second level supervisor?

In particular these two males have the responsibility of stimulating the libido of a large group of both female and male employees in a large retail company. These two particular males seem to be aggressive and threatening when they approach me in particular (one reason being I do not display my sexuality openly or in a threatening manner and therefore find it distasteful when this occurs to me).

These supervisors have the authority to fire the employees and I wish to bond with them in an upwardly-mobile way. Are there any hints that you can suggest to help me communicate/bond with these men in both a physical and verbal way? I do stimulate libido with my voice but not physically. Maybe I should. In what way could I do so without appearing to mimick or insult the "horny toad" population of the workforce?

Sincerely,
Subordinate worker>>

⊠⊠⊠

Dear Subordinate,

It is not completely clear to me what it means when you write, "...these two males have the responsibility of stimulating the libido of a large group of both female and male employees..." That is suggestive of a form of sexual harassment in the workplace. There are state and federal laws against sexual harassment, and it should not occur in the workplace, school, church, or anywhere else where there are supervisors or authority figures who may take unfair advantage of subordinates.

You did not state whether you are a male or female — and your letter could have been written by either. In either case, the laws against sexual harassment in the workplace would apply.

If you feel that this is not really a case of sexual harassment, but rather more a matter of learning how to get along with the different personality styles of your supervisors, I would recommend a more standard effort to get to know them, greet them with ease and confidence, always listen to what they have to say and give the impression that you appreciate their thoughts and supervision.

Under no circumstances should you emulate the openly sexual, physically and verbally aggressive style that you find threatening and distasteful yourself.

If you know an employee who has been there for a long time, someone around whom you feel comfortable, talk to that person and find out how they handle their relationship with these supervisors. You can learn a lot from the veteran employees.

Good luck, and thanks for writing.

⊠⊠⊠

<<Dr. Roth. Thank you for the reply. I'll use my one-minute friendliness techniques and try to not be offended by different opinions regarding office standard behavior. Unfortunately I am aware, even if I was sexually harrassed, I would have to prove so in court. The compensation would not be great, and the chances of

finding another job would be considerably narrowed! Thank you more for the moral support!>>

⊠⊠⊠

You are very welcome.
Best wishes, and thanks for writing.

⊠⊠⊠

Criminal Profiling

<< Dear Dr. Roth,

My son is entering eleventh grade and is interested in forensics. He is interested in understanding the psychology of a criminal in hopes of determining his innocence or guilt. He called it "criminal profiling." Would this be called forensic psychology or behavioral forensics or what? What is an approximate salary and is it a job that most like who enter this field? Thank you very much for taking time from your busy schedule.

Lizzie>>

✉✉✉

Dear Lizzie,

There are many ways to enter the field of criminal profiling. One might start with a degree in Psychology, and enter specialized training areas from there. This can also be done by psychiatrists, but that requires a desire to go through medical school first.

One might also begin in the Criminal Justice field, and from there receive specialized training in psychology. I am sending you a link which may be helpful in providing you with additional resources:

American Board of Forensic Psychology
http://www.abfp.com/

Also, be sure to check the "Frequently Asked Questions" section on my web page.

With respect to salaries, they vary considerably. Income in the private sector tends to exceed that of salaried government employees, such as in police departments.

Best wishes to you and your son, and thanks for writing.

✉✉✉

Depends on Hearing the Hard Rap Music

<< Dear Dr. Roth:

My son has been diagnosed as Paranoid Schizophrenia but he will not take medication or see a Psychiatrist. He seems to have mood swings only with me. He functions well but seems to be super-obsessed with and depends upon hearing the hard rap music. He writes constantly and I look over his writings without him knowing and there are things that just don't meet reality. I don't know what to do and I am constantly praying that God will relieve him of this situation.

He is 27 years old, has had two years of college. I had to bring him home from college 5 years ago. He went through many changes from receiving a horrified treatment in the hospital emergency room to living on the streets in his car during the summer. He presently lives at his aunt's house. He is not well, but he will not accept any help because he is convinced he is beating this, but he is not.

He seems all right but has mood swings where he feels I am bothering him. Is there someone or somewhere I can get help. I have a hospital plan and whatever I can do to help, I will do because I want my son to be well. He is my only child, and I am a divorced parent.

Please give me help, I have not had any luck with anyone or anybody reaching him.

Have a BLESSED CHRISTMAS

Thank you
Colleen M.>>

⊠ ⊠ ⊠

Dear Colleen,

You have one of the most difficult jobs in the world — parenting an emotionally or mentally ill child who is an adult. The very first thing I would advise you to do is to check out the following:

National Alliance for the Mentally Ill
http://www.nami.org/

This organization will be able to offer you both advice and support. They have been helping parents and other relatives of mentally ill children and adults since 1979.

The difficult part of parenting is "letting go" — letting your child be the adult he has become. Recognizing that you no longer have control over your child, and shouldn't have, because he is no longer a child, is the ultimate milestone in parenting. When your adult-child is mentally ill, that takes on a dimension of difficulty beyond what any parent can imagine, who does not have a mentally ill child.

Your son is still an adult, and you must recognize that and treat him as such. These are the most telling sentences in your letter: "He is not well, but he will not accept any help because he is convinced he is beating this, but he is not ... He seems all right but has mood swings where he feels I am bothering him..."

You may not realize that those sentiments may be felt by any parent of any adult child who is going through any problem in his or her life. It is very important that they try to do it themselves; to be allowed to manage their lives and their problems like any adult; to be treated as an adult by their own parents.

If you take that away from your son — no matter that you are trying to help him and to keep him out of harm's way — he will resent you for it. That is actually normal! Your son needs to find his own way because that is the only way he will accept. You must respect his wishes as an adult. Otherwise, he will grow to resent you and you will not be helping him at all.

Your son may need to find out for himself that he has to take his meds or suffer the consequences, such as more "horrified" treatment experiences in hospitals and emergency rooms, over and over. The treatment can surely seem horrific to the patient who may need to be restrained to prevent him from hurting himself or others in the midst of a florid psychosis. Sometimes we have to let our loved ones find things out for themselves and come to their own conclusions.

As long as your son is resentful of your attempts to guide him, you cannot guide him. Let him try as best he can to guide himself. That is so much easier said than done, but that is what you have to do – let him know that you are there if and when he needs you. Otherwise, wait in the wings.

Your signature suggests that you are a religious person. This is the time to have faith. Good luck to you and your son, and thanks for writing.

✉✉✉

Max Salary

<< I have a question about starting salary. I live in Orlando Florida and I plan on majoring in forensic psychology. I would like to know the Max salary that I could make. Eli>>

⊠⊠⊠

Dear Eli,

Salary depends on where you work — privately, or for an institution. You may look over the "Frequently Asked Questions" section of my web page. I am also forwarding another link to you which may help answer your questions:

American Board of Forensic Psychology
http://www.abfp.com/

Good luck and thanks for writing.

⊠⊠⊠

Desperately Needs Geriatric Psychiatrist

<< Hi Dr Roth,

I found your web site and in desperation, am hoping you can advise me....My 87-yr-old mother <u>desperately needs</u> a GERIATRIC psychiatrist, and also, a GERIATRIC neurologist. Otherwise, normal practicing doctors just are not that interested in an 87-year-old!

Could you please recommend for the New York City area and/or refer me to who could direct us to those doctors??? No Medical Society I call can and neither can any doctor I ask here!

Thanks you so much,
Millie>>

⊠⊠⊠

Dear Millie,

I found the following information at this website:

American Association of Geriatric Psychiatry
http://www.aagpgpa.org/

"AAGP can provide the names (2-3) of Board Certified Geriatric Psychiatrists in your geographic area or the geographic area of someone about whom you care. Email main@aagponline.org *and include your name as well as the city and zip code for the*

area in which you would like to see a doctor. We will email you contact information promptly."

Please be sure that anyone you are referred to is Board Certified and in good standing with the State Board of Professional Standards.

Best wishes, and thanks for writing.

✉✉✉

Sexual Side Effects

<<Dear Dr. Roth,

I have two questions, which I really hope you can help me with!

The first question regards the sexual side effects of SSRI's [Selective Serotonin Reuptake Inhibitors, a class of anti-depressant medication]. I have been on them for the past 3 years (switched from Prozac to Zoloft, then Celexa). The dosages I took for each were average (not high). I had no sexual difficulties at all prior to starting them 3 years ago — in fact, I'd say I was sexually robust. While on them, I definitely experienced sexual side effects (loss of libido, loss of blood flow, no or poor climax).

I have not been on any SSRI's for almost 2 months now (mainly because I couldn't stand the sexual side effects anymore), and yet I still have some sexual difficulties, though not quite as bad as when I was actually on them. (I'm now on Wellbutrin). My question is, have the 3 years that I used SSRI's permanently damaged my sexual libido/capacity? Can I ever expect it to return? And if so, will it be as strong as before, or weakened?

Also, I have been on Wellbutrin for the past 3 weeks, but now want to get off it as I'm experiencing jitteriness and dry mouth. I'm taking 150 mg. per day right now. I understand that side effects are common when first starting a new medication, but this has been going on for just over 3 weeks now. Also, my doctor initially suggested I go to 300 mg. a day, and I don't see that happening as I can barely handle 150 mg. a day.

My second question is, what meds do you recommend (for mild depression) that do not have sexual OR jittery side effects? For example, I have read a bit about Serzone and Remeron.

Thank you so much for your help! I hope you will be able to answer soon. Please reply directly to me by email (please don't publish my letter on any public forum), and please do not use my name or email address publicly. Thanks.

Anonymous Female.>>

⊠⊠⊠

Dear Anonymous,

I would not use your name or e-mail address in any publication. All of the names in this book are changed. Your letter is one of so many which I receive asking about side effects of medications — frequently sexual side effects — that I could publish any one of them and you could not tell if it were yours!

Wellbutrin (bupropion) is commonly substituted for SSRI's when they cause the sexual side effects that you describe, so that, too, would not in any way identify you. Moreover, if your name did not accompany your e-mail, I could not be sure if it were written by a male or female, as I have received letters such as yours from both — but many more from men than women.

Once you stopped the SSRI's for a few weeks, your libido, or sexual desire, should have returned to normal. I can say with a high degree of certainty that there has been no permanent damage in that regard. The reason you are still having some trouble may be because the Wellbutrin is not treating your depression adequately, and suppression of libido is a common symptom of depression; or your psychological worry or anxiety over whether your libido would return to normal is itself reducing your libido. This latter problem is a frequent cause of male impotence (erectile failure). In other words, just worrying about it can cause the problem itself. It is also possible that you need to give your libido a little more time to normalize. Three weeks is not a very long time for this purpose.

The jitteriness and dry mouth you are experiencing from the Wellbutrin may indicate the dose is too high for you. Wellbutrin can be given in doses as low as 37.5mg (1/2 of a 75mg tablet) once or twice a day. If it is working to keep your depression in check, you may be able to <u>gradually</u> reduce the dose, maintain the benefit and lose the side effects.

If gradually reducing the dose does not help, it would dictate that you try another medication. There are more than two dozen antidepressants on the market. One may work very well in alleviating depression for one person but not another; and one person may experience side effects but not someone else. So it is worth trying others. There are simply too many antidepressants on the market, old and new, to stay with one or another that is causing problems.

Newer medications usually have their own sets of side effects. You may certainly try them, but don't eschew the older ones. The research literature may suggest that the newer meds have "better side effect profiles," but that depends on how each individual is affected. The older meds are worth trying if the new ones are not doing the job.

Good luck to you, and thanks for writing.

✉✉✉

Single Mom Looking for a Career

<< Hi my name is Francine and I am a 19-year-old single mom looking for a career. I am interested in so many different fields such as nursing, ob-gyn, law, forensics, and psychiatry. I am really afraid that I am going to go through school and hate whatever career I choose and be stuck in it.

Finally I narrowed it down and I decided that I was going to go to college and major in criminology and biology. I am smart but I goofed off a lot in high school. I have matured a lot since then and I would really love to pursue a career dealing with criminals, but as a doctor. I do not want to be a police officer. So I guess to get to my question is there any way to redeem myself for the mistakes I have made as a child. I am willing to do whatever it takes.

I am interested in so many different fields and I just know that there is a career out there that has to do with them all. Please help me any way you can.
Thank You,
Francine>>

⊠⊠⊠

Dear Francine,

You might sign up for some community college courses in the areas where you can show — and see for yourself — what your actual capabilities are. Take some first-level courses in a wide variety of subjects, such as humanities, mathematics and the sciences. If you do well in those, continue to take increasingly higher level studies.

Take a small load at first, and see what you can do. If you can show good work in your courses now, the higher level schools you apply to in the future would likely acknowledge that and give it more weight than earlier work in high school which may have been substandard.

Best wishes and thanks for writing.

✉✉✉

True Love: Definition

<< Hi. I'm writing a feature story for my high school newspaper on "True Love." What is your definition of it, and can it happen with teenagers? I understand that you don't specialize in this area but any help or input you could give me I would really appreciate.

1. What is your definition of "true love"?

2. How is a person to know they are in love? (Are there actual signs or symptoms you can see?)

3. "Teenagers can fall in true love." How do you feel about that statement?

Well, those are it. If you could just answer them, I would greatly appreciate it.

Thanks
Flower Baby>>

⊠⊠⊠

Dear FlowerBaby,
Those are difficult questions because "love" means different things to different people. "Narcissus" was a mythical character who fell in love with his own reflection in a pond and fell in trying to grasp it. He drowned. That is the background for the advice that warns us against being too "narcissistic." (And

unfortunately, it is sometimes difficult to distinguish between healthy self-esteem and unhealthy narcissism.)

Love must be more than attraction & longing. An alcoholic "loves" alcohol, but that is different from the loving bond between two human beings. The difference resides in a willingness to sacrifice. *True love includes a desire to see the other person happy — even when that requires* letting them go.

The Biblical story of King Solomon and the two new mothers is the best example: Two women each gave birth to a baby on the same day. That night, one of the babies died. When the mother realized that her baby was dead, she waited for the other mother to fall asleep, and switched the babies. When the other mother awoke, she immediately knew what happened. She wanted her baby returned — but the first mother insisted that the live baby was hers.

King Solomon was asked to mediate. He said, "It is only fair that I cut the baby in half and give each mother half." He raised his sword over his head and prepared to strike the infant.

The mother whose baby had died said nothing.

The child's real mother raised her arms up to shield him and said, "Do not harm my baby!! Give him to the other woman!!" *That* willingness to sacrifice her own child *in order to save its life revealed the real mother. King Solomon returned the baby to her. She showed true love.*

Therefore, in answer to your first question, my definition of "true love" is: A willingness to sacrifice — even to give up a loved one — in order to insure the loved one's happiness.

Your second question is a little tricky. The initial clue that one may be "in love" is usually a physical attraction; a strong desire to be around the other person. Signs and symptoms include thinking about the other person frequently, even when they are not around; and feeling nervous or anxious — but especially exhuberant and happy — when they are around.

Sexual attraction, though, is not the same as love. It can turn into love, when the additional criteria are added. That means, not only a desire to be around that person, and a willingness to sacrifice for that person's happiness, but also a reciprocal feeling from the other person. Love is a dynamic, "living" thing. It requires food and nurturance, or it shrinks and dies — just like all living things. When love is not reciprocated — when it is a one-way street — it will eventually starve and wither away. That is similar to the attraction we have to our favorite movie stars. We "love" them, and we "sacrifice" our time and our money to buy tickets to see them — but it is not the same as "true love" at all. There is no reciprocity.

With respect to your third question — can teenagers fall in "true love" — yes. Some teenagers even get married, have children, live together for forty or fifty years, and never stop loving and sacrificing for each other. The reciprocity and willingness to sacrifice *for each other is the key.*

I hope you find this helpful. Good luck in your studies, and thanks for writing.

◻◻◻

Can't Stop Checking

<< Every night before I go to sleep I check on my kids to make sure they are okay. I look around the house to make sure everything looks fine. When I finally lay down it takes me around 30 min. to an hour before I can shut my eyes. All these thoughts keep going through my head that something is going to happen as soon as I close my eyes. I keep thinking what if the house catches on fire and we can't get out. Or somebody might break in the house and me, my husband and my 6 month old twins can get out safely, and my 6 year old can't. He has his own room and I keep thinking that I won't be able to help him if something happens. If I hear a bark, or branches hitting the house I get scared and I can't go back to sleep. I get up and check around the house to make sure everything is okay at least three times during the night. Then the next day I'm tired and I'm worn out but I have to get up for my twins. I do this every night. If I forget to check on something before I lay down, I have to get up or I can't go to sleep and my heart will start racing thinking something's going to happen. Am I stupid or a psycho. I'm embarassed to tell a doctor for fear that they'll laugh at me.

Sincerely, Giselle>>

⊠⊠⊠

Dear Giselle,

There are several possible conditions that your symptoms describe. With 6-month-old twins, it is possible – even likely – that you are suffering from a post-partum depression. Symptoms can include depression, anxiety – and in more severe cases, paranoid thoughts, or even hallucinations or delusions.

Alternatively, the description of "all these thoughts going through my head" keeping you from falling asleep may be the "racing thoughts" of a manic or hypo- (just below) -manic condition. Such symptoms can be triggered in post-partum women who may be predisposed to bipolar disorder, or have family members with bipolar traits.

Another possible diagnosis is obsessive - compulsive disorder (OCD), the hallmark of which is the constant need to "check" things, along with a constant feeling of anxiety that things are not settled, or not secure; hence the need to keep checking over and over again.

A psychiatrist should be consulted to do a thorough psychiatric evaluation to identify the correct diagnosis and prescribe medication that can help you obtain relief from your symptoms. A psychiatrist can collaborate with your Ob-gyn doctor to run appropriate tests to determine if there is something else that may be causing your symptoms.

Psychotherapy for postpartum emotional disorders can also be extremely helpful. A licensed psychologist, psychiatric nurse practitioner or clinical social worker can help in the evaluation and treatment of your symptoms.

For more information, below is a link which you might find helpful:

National Institutes of Mental Health(NIMH)
Postpartum Depression
http://www.nlm.nih.gov/medlineplus/postpartumdepression.html

Best wishes and thanks for writing.

✉✉✉

I Want To Be A Songwriter

<<Hi Dr. Roth, I want to thank you ahead of time if you read and respond to this message. I read through your website and wanted to ask you a question though. I'll try to be brief.

I'm 23 years old, with a B.A. [Bachelor of Arts] degree from the University of Maryland in English Literature, minor in Art. I want to be a songwriter in life (it is just a passion for me), but career-wise, frankly, I'm apathetic towards the "corporate world," and after working in government I've become disenchanted with it — I realized the stereotypes about politics are unfortunately very true, and I had to get out.

Psychology and Psychiatry have always been career fields in the back of my mind that I never pursued. Why? Frankly, I hated math, I was terrible at it, so I just started to shy away from the sciences and instead towards liberal arts. I took an accounting course my freshman year in college, and I just hated it. So I ended up with literature and art in college because it was easy for me. After all, I wanted to be a musician. I *was* interested in biology and psychology, however. I enjoyed my science courses in high school and psychology courses in college.

So my question is this: Is it too late for me to pursue a career in psychiatry? I understand it takes many many years of education and training. I'm just wondering if my choices in college will make me "behind the field," so to speak, when trying to enter medical school. I'm thinking I should initially take some undergraduate courses at a local college to see if the science aspect is interesting to me — to see if I can really get into it, like I got into music for example. Should I pursue a full B.S. [Bachelor of Science] degree?

It's just a nagging thought I've always had, and I wanted some advice from a professional in the field.

Well, thanks a million, I know this wasn't quite "brief," but I appreciate your patience and any thoughts you might have. Thanks again,
Ken>>

⊠⊠⊠

Dear Ken,

Since I did not go to college until I was 27, I would say it is not "too late" for you to pursue anything that interests you. Psychiatry is a medical specialty, and in order to get into medical school, and to get through it, you do have to take higher level math courses, such as trigonometry, analytic geometry, and calculus. It is possible to study hard, get some tutoring when necessary, and pass those courses.

I only want to warn you that you will find "stereotypes" in the medical world — not just in politics — and everywhere else. If you love what you do, you have to accept, and work around, people who are not necessarily committed to good work and ethical values in life. And you will find them everywhere you go.

Best wishes and thanks for writing.

⊠⊠⊠

<<Wow, thanks a lot for your answer, it helps a lot, honestly. Take care and good luck to you as well,
Ken>>

My Sister Has a Psychiatric Disorder

<<Dear Dr. Roth,

I have a younger sister, age 46 who has a major psychiatric disorder. She goes in and out of being very paranoid. She thinks people are doing things to her and they're not. For example, she thinks someone is coming into her apartment and putting stool on her floor or urinating on her carpet. She thinks people are talking about her, or tapping her phone. She closes herself in her apartment, drawing all curtains and sometime not coming out for 1 or 2 months.

What's worse, she doesn't think anything is wrong with her. She is starting to hate us (her brothers and sisters) when we ask to take her for help. Also, she will go off and hear someone talking to her, and she answers who she hears. She talks to herself and answers herself in a different tone of voice. That is real scary.

We at this point are lost. She is not harming herself in any way, which we were told, gives her the right to choose not to go and seek help. She was earlier diagnosed as a Skits-a-frinic (I probably didn't spell it correctly). But we think there is more to this diagnosis. Her medicine isn't working. Can you please tell us what you think, or what can we do to help her?

Kassie>>

⊠⊠⊠

Dear Kassie,

Your sister has all the signs and symptoms for a diagnosis of schizophrenia. It is not common to have the disorder initially at age 46, though — it usually has its onset in the teen years or very early 20's.

If your sister was healthy, normally friendly and sociable, and did not have any of the symptoms you described recently in her life, such as 20's or 30's, then she could be suffering from another type of illness. This could be Bipolar Disorder or even Post-partum Psychosis, if it began after giving birth. There are other possible causes, such as drug or alcohol abuse. Some illicit drugs such as cocaine and marijuana are known to cause paranoid delusions in some users. Legally prescribed drugs can also be abused and cause some of the symptoms. Initially, though, a physical cause in the brain tissue itself needs to be ruled-out. Your sister should have a complete medical/physical examination. She can start with her own family physician, internal medicine physician, or neurologist. All possible causes should be examined that may account for your sister's symptoms and/or changes in mental status.

You cannot force your sister to seek treatment, unless, as you have already discovered, she is saying or doing things which could be harmful to herself or others. If that is the case, then you can seek a commitment petition to have her taken to a psychiatric facility for examination. This would be done through your family doctor or local law enforcement agency.

Needless to say, the commitment process would not endear you to your sister, but would possibly cause a worsening of the relationship, with even less trust on her part. That is why it is best not to go this route unless she is clearly endangering herself or others. The best way to deal with your sister, if there is no dangerous behavior, is to keep in contact, and let her know that you love and support her, and that you are ready to help whenever she feels she needs help.

One particularly good organization which you might find very helpful is the following:

National Alliance for the Mentally Ill (NAMI)
http://www.nami.org/

Good luck, and thanks for writing.

⊠⊠⊠

Depression or Not Wanting to Grow Up

<< Dear Dr. Roth...

I am searching for a psychiatrist specializing in Child and Adolescent issues in the St. Louis area. My soon-to-be-stepdaughter lives with my fiancé and me, and he (her father) has had no luck in finding a good therapist for her. She has not responded to any treaments nor different forms of medication.

At issue is whether her behavior is really depression or not wanting to grow up and take responsibility. I realize that only a trained professional can assess this, but to date, not one of the 3 different therapists or 2 psychiatrists seem to have helped her. Her behavior has not changed, even though she has been on 3 different types of medication (Paxil, Zoloft and now Effexor).

She does use drugs (LSD, Ecstasy and pot), but she said she doesn't use them regularly. My research indicates that all of these are mind-altering and can cause personality changes. We are just helpless to help her. She won't get up before 2:00 every day, won't go to school, and every job she has had (2) she only goes to work for a few days a week then gets fired.

I realize that there is much, much more you would need to know but I am hoping that you can refer us to a really good CHILD & ADOLESCENT PSYCHIATRIST here. She has only been to women, and she doesn't really respond well to women. I am thinking we need to try a man therapist this time — anything to help.

Thanks so much for taking the time to read this, and hopefully, you can guide us.
Rachel >>

⊠⊠⊠

Dear Rachel,

You did not say how old your step-daughter is. I am assuming she is in her late teens or early 20's. People who use LSD, "ecstasy" (MDMA, a synthetic drug chemically similar to both methamphetamine and the hallucinogen mescaline) and smoke pot (marijuana), will continue to have problems until they abstain from drug use (although there is flourishing debate about marijuana[1]).

It may be that your fiancé's daughter is using drugs because she is depressed or otherwise mentally disturbed; but the drugs are exacerbating the condition. (You did not mention alcohol, but that, too, can be very destructive, especially in combination with the other substances.) Your first job is to get her clean and sober. Until that occurs, she is unlikely to benefit from any psychotherapy or medication.

In the meantime, you and her father should attend counseling yourselves, specifically to help you learn how to deal with your daughter's problems. She may have to go to a drug rehabilitation clinic, and through counseling you can learn how to go about making that happen.

Some resources which you can check out include the following: American Academy of Child and Adolescent Psychiatry, where you can find a board-certified psychiatrist in your area. Also, the National Alliance for the Mentally Ill is a family group which helps people deal with mentally disturbed family members. The Al-Anon/Alateen group can provide a lot of support and

---

[1] Advocates of legalizing marijuana claim that it is "relaxing" or "mellows them out." There are medical uses for marijuana, or *cannabis*, including reduction of intra-ocular pressure in glaucoma patients, reduction of nausea from chemotherapy, and increasing the appetite in patients with AIDS and other "wasting" disorders. However, marijuana can trigger psychotic symptoms, especially paranoia, in people predisposed to such conditions. Given that our Presidents, two Presidents before him, and one Vice-President have all admitted to smoking marijuana, it would seem that de-criminalization, at least, is just.

guidance for you and your husband, as they work with those who have family members that drink or use drugs :

National Alliance for the Mentally Ill (NAMI)
http://www.nami.org/

American Academy of Child and Adolescent Psychiatry
http://www.aacap.org/

Al-Anon/Alateen
http://www.al-anon.alateen.org/

Above all, I encourage you to continue to be supportive and loving, and avoid chiding her, or suggesting that she needs to grow up, or that she is shirking responsibility. Those admonishments almost never accomplish the desired goal, and often have the opposite effect. Let her know you love her, and avoid any judgmental or critical comments. Continue to help her look for help if she wants it. She must desire the help to make use of it. That will take time, but eventually will pay off.

Good luck, and thanks for writing.

✉ ✉ ✉

Why Math & Science?

<<Hello,

I am a 14 year old and interested in psychiatry. We started a school project and we need to research it. I chose psychiatry. I was reading on the internet on your website, and it said I needed a lot of math and science. I was just wondering why you would need math and science for psychiatry?

Thanks, Lawrence>>

⊠⊠⊠

Dear Lawrence,

Psychiatry is a medical specialty, and you need lots of math and science to get into (and through) medical school. You have to be able to understand physiological processes such as blood pressure, medication dosing, the chemistry of disease processes and the metabolism of drugs.

Psychiatrists must be able to understand these things in order to examine their patients correctly, prescribe medications such as antidepressants and tranquilizers accurately and safely; and to diagnose psychiatric disorders that may be the result of other medical diseases.

Good luck in your studies, and thanks for writing.

⊠⊠⊠

Abusive Boyfriend

<<I am in an abusive relationship and I am deathly afraid. He has already told me that if I try to leave him that he will kill me. Actually he has already threaten to kill me several times. He is doing something to my mind. I don't want to eat, I can't sleep at night, I just feel depressed and alone most of the time. I can't talk to anyone else about this. What should I do?
Lucille>>

⊠⊠⊠

Dear Lucille,

You should go to the police and file a report. If not, then your boyfriend may eventually make good on his threats. He may threaten that things will get worse if you go to the police, but if you do not *go to the police, things* are bound to get worse. *You must file formal charges and* follow through *with the charges, attending every hearing, and sticking to the facts. Do not drop the charges, as that will only bring things back to the way they are now.*

Get professional help to find out why you allowed yourself to enter and remain in this abusive relationship. Often there is a "repetition" of such relationships, as the subconscious keeps hoping things will some day turn out differently. You need to get help to understand why you are attracted to this person, in spite of red flags and warning signs.

Have faith in yourself and the fact that you do not deserve to be abused – no one does – and, yes, things really can be better.

Good luck, and thanks for writing.

⊠⊠⊠

<< This morning when me and my boyfriend had an agrument, he didn't hit when I was yelling at him, like he usually does. Is that a sign? Lucille >>

⊠⊠⊠

Dear Lucille,

That may be a sign that he was not feeling well. It is also a sign that you understand the "triggers" in your relationship, such as yelling at your boyfriend. It sounds as though you <u>expected</u> your yelling to trigger his physical abuse, yet you were unable to stop yourself.

It is very important that you get help to understand why you remain in this repetitive cycle of trigger/abuse/trigger/abuse. Please talk to your family doctor about seeing a psychiatrist. If there is a mental health clinic in your county, that is a good place to get help without costing a lot.

⊠⊠⊠

<< Me and my b/f have not spoken to each other since yesterday. How can I make him leave without him getting angry or violent. I just want to get out of this relationship alive and not have to worry about him coming back and trying to do something to me.
Lucille >>

⊠⊠⊠

Dear Lucille,

It seems that your relationship with your boyfriend takes a circular path — Anger is triggered, yelling begins, then physical abuse, then not speaking. It is very common for dysfunctional relationships to display a clear pattern like that. The pattern of your relationship suggests that eventually your boyfriend will become violent again.

You should, as I originally said, go to the police and file charges. However, if you choose to remain with your boyfriend and cannot bring yourself to make the move to extricate yourself from this relationship safely, than the first step is to find a licensed certified counselor. This could be a clergyman, a psychologist, a psychiatrist, a licensed clinical social worker, or a psychiatric nurse practitioner. Preferably they should be skilled in marriage or couple's counseling. You should go to the counselor first, yourself, and explain the situation. Then ask your boyfriend to join you. Tell him that the cycle of anger, yelling, hitting, and then not speaking, needs to be broken.

If your boyfriend is reluctant to go, tell him that going to a counselor is a very small commitment to help avoid your relationship ending with one or both of you seriously injured or killed. You must insist on his joining you, but if he won't then you must go yourself. Your counselor should be able to help you extricate yourself from this relationship and also determine why you may be attracted to destructive, painful relationships.

Best of luck to you.

⊠⊠⊠

<< I agree, I do need to seek professional help and so does he. I have told him this many times. This weekend he found out that I lied to him since the beginning of our relationship and he went crazy, he said that he was going to kill me. He took me to a canal and he said that he was going to push me off, but when we got there he couldn't do it. He just cried, he said no matter how mad I make him or how much he wants to do it, he said he just can't. How do I convince him to come with me to get some help? Who do I call to

get help? I don't have a lot of money, but I do want the help. We both need it. Lucille>>

⊠⊠⊠

Dear Lucille,

Look in the white pages of the phone book under your County Health or Mental Health services. You can also look in the yellow pages under "Clinics" — but be sure that you are going to a legitimate clinic with certified, licensed practitioners.

If there is a medical school near you, or a hospital affiliated with a university, they frequently offer counseling services on a sliding scale.

Good luck to you both.

⊠⊠⊠

<< Thank you, I will do that and I will keep you informed on how everything is going. Thanks for being there when I really needed someone to talk to.
Lucille>>

⊠⊠⊠

You are very welcome.

⊠⊠⊠

<<This morning he told me that he is going to give me what I want. He said that he is going home today. I'm not getting my hopes up until he actually leaves. Just pray that he goes through with it and leaves.
Lucille>>

⊠⊠⊠

I am praying, Lucille.

⊠⊠⊠

<<No, everything did not go well. I feel like I'm at my last rope. I just can't take it anymore, I realize now that he is not going to change. I hate myself for allowing this to happen to me. He is a liar and I just feel so depressed right now that I feel like crying.
Lucille>>

⊠⊠⊠

Dear Lucille,

I'm sorry to hear that — but not surprised. You should begin to identify the pattern now — the cycle of abuse. You must talk to a professional, as I recommended previously. You did not say whether your boyfriend is hitting you, but if so, you should go to the police. There may even be a clinical social worker with the police dept. who may be able to help you.

Best of luck to you both.

⊠⊠⊠

Getting Licensed

<<Hello. I am curious to see how I would go about getting licensed to practice psychotherapy in New Jersey. I have a four year degree from an accredited college. I majored in psycholgy/sociology. I do not want to become a psychiatrist, only a psychotherapist. Thank you for your time.

Tim

⊠⊠⊠

Dear Tim,
*   Below is the link to the American Psychotherapy Association. You may be able to ask them about the qualifications for licensure in N. J.:*

American Psychotherapy Association
http://www.americanpsychotherapy.com/

Good luck, and thanks for writing.

⊠⊠⊠

Donate Organs for Cash?

<<hello how are you?
how can i donate organs for cash?
B.B.>>

⊠⊠⊠

Dear B. B.:

There is an ongoing debate regarding the issue of allowing people to sell their organs for cash, rather than donating them without any compensation. Selling one's organs is an acceptable practice in some countries, but is illegal in the United States. Since 1984, there has been a federal law in effect with a $50,000 penalty for engaging in the sale of organs for profit. The issue is still hotly debated in research and medical forums, however. The essence of the debate is as follows:

If organs are sold for profit, then the poorest of the poor will be selling theirs, while only the rich would be able to buy organs and have the transplant they need.

On the other hand, if donors were paid for donating organs, the lists of organ transplant recipients could disappear or be drastically reduced. For example, according to the United Network for Organ Sharing (UNOS), as of December, 2008, more than 100,000 candidates were awaiting organ donations; but for the first nine months of 2008, only about 20,000 organs were transplanted, from about 10,000 individual donors.

You may visit the UNOS website, or the Organ Procurement and Transplantation Network (OPTN) website for more information:

United Network for Organ Sharing
http://www.UNOS.org

Organ Procurement and Transplantation Network
http://www.OPTN.org/

I hope you find this information helpful.

⊠⊠⊠

<<Thanks for your help. I haven't had any luck yet but I won't give up. I hear that there's a place in Galveston that was taking organs for cash but I still haven't located it yet. My husband wants to donate one of his testicles so I'm trying to help him out. Thanks for your help, I appreciate it sincerely. B. B.>>

⊠⊠⊠

Dear B. B.:

I do not know of any place in Galveston that would purchase organs. Moreover, I am not aware that testicles can be transplanted — only kidney, liver, pancreas, heart, lung, intestines, and corneas.

I suggest that you speak with a psychiatrist in your area. If you live in Texas, contact your local county agency for a doctor who might be able to see you on a sliding scale fee basis.

⊠⊠⊠

Future for Psychiatry?

<<Dear Dr. Roth,

1. What do you believe the Future outlook is for Psychiatry? 5 – 10 years from now.
2. What is the most Challenging Thing you find in psychiatry?
3. What are some good Schools Offering Programs in Psychiatry?

These Questions are for a Report, And I need Help, Thank you for time

Debbie.>>

⊠⊠⊠

Dear Debbie,

1. Emotional problems, substance abuse, and behavioral problems will always be with us. For that reason, psychiatry will always be needed. The majority of medical students have primary interests in other areas, such as internal medicine or surgery. There are never enough medical doctors to fill all of the psychiatry training programs. We need to promote more interest in the field.

2. The most challenging thing for me is to make the correct diagnosis and prescribe the correct medication for each patient.

3. There are many residency programs in psychiatry, but first it is necessary to complete college and then medical school. By that

time, you will have more of an idea about where you want to apply for psychiatric residency training.

Good luck to you in the future, and thanks for writing.

✉✉✉

Oppositional and Defiant

<< Dear Dr. Roth, My daughter has been diagnosed with "Oppositional Defiant Disorder," and she has ADHD with Hyperactivity. I'm not sure, but I think she is Compulsive, Impulsive, and Defiant. She takes no medicine and she has no counseling.

When she was younger she would pick holes in her head. She is 28 now and has a daughter. Sometimes she takes care of her daughter very well, but if she takes a notion, she doesn't take care of her at all. She is a chronic liar, and she will steal. She has never been able to keep a friend or boyfriend. Her child's father is a fourteen-year-old boy.

Our whole family has tried to help her, with her kid and with herself. Now there's a chance that she may lose the kid, but we are going to do everything to keep her. The problem is, "How can we get her into a hospital or on medication?" She won't do it herself. We need some advice. Thank You.
Queenie>>

⊠⊠⊠

Dear Queenie:

The diagnoses you mentioned, such as Oppositional Defiant Disorder, are usually diagnosed in children. If your daughter is stealing and failing to care for her child, she might be diagnosed as an Antisocial Personality Disorder. But she may have more serious psychiatric problems, such as bipolar disorder or schizophrenia. In any case, she must live up to her legal obligations if she is able to understand them.

You stated that your daughter may lose custody of her child and you hope to keep her. Family members are often considered the first choice as a foster home placement in the event that a child is removed from their parent. You may want to discuss this with the social service agency that is involved, expressing your concern and offering your help.

If your daughter is unwilling to get help, often the social service agencies will require and arrange it for her. I recommend that you also find a family therapist to go to yourself, and then perhaps bring your daughter into the therapy. In the meantime, it is important that you let your daughter know that you love her, and will always support her emotionally, but you cannot help her if she will not get professional help and follow her doctor's advice.

Good luck, and thanks for writing.

✉✉✉

Note-taking and Record-keeping

<<Dear Dr. Roth:

I intend to open a private practice in general psychiatry soon in Western Massachusetts and wonder if you have any suggestions as to how I might expedite my note-taking and record-keeping. For example, do you use any forms that could be helpful? Have you any experience using a palm pilot as a note-generating device? Thank you in advance for your help.

Sincerely,
A.S., MD >>

⊠⊠⊠

Dear Dr. A.S.,

I do not have a Palm Pilot, so I do not know how that would work. I still take notes the old-fashioned way — jotting down a few key words and dates. If I am at a computer, I type the notes as we talk. If you can do that, and your patient does not mind, it is ideal.

When interviewing a patient, it is important that you spend most of the time having good eye contact. Regardless of how intently you may be listening, people tend to feel somewhat "brushed aside" if you continually look down at your notes – or keyboard – and not up at them.

Good luck in your new practice, and thanks for writing.

⊠⊠⊠

Swiss Cheese Memory

For years now (since my early teens) I have been living with frustrating short and long term memory problems, which also includes problems with word recall. I don't remember movies I've watched, books I've read, places I've been, etc. It's as if I live in the present all the time. Word recall is the worst — I am constantly using the wrong word to describe an object or action.

I have been taking meds for ADD and Depression for two years. However, the memory lapses have always been consistent before, during and after diagnosis, treatment and therapy. I consider myself to be a pretty well-adjusted, "normal" 27-year-old female. I know stress can play a role in memory problems associated with depression, however I am an at-home mom with a loving, supportive husband. Even my psychiatrist can't explain why these lapses and recall problems have been consistent and do not respond to medication/therapy. ANY IDEAS? My kids think I'm a walking Mrs. Magoo!>>

⊠⊠⊠

Dear Mrs. Magoo,

You did not say whether you have been examined by a neurologist (specialist in disorders of the nervous system), but if not, then you should do so. You can get a referral from your family physician or from your psychiatrist. This is a fairly unusual problem to have without evidence of either a traumatic brain injury, seizure disorder, or medication side effect. On the other hand, it may be something more akin to a learning disorder or learning disability. A psychologist who conducts psychological-educational testing may be able to help diagnose the problem. Your psychiatrist should be able to make a referral to a psychologist who can conduct the proper testing.

Some medications, such as benzodiazepines (Valium, Librium, Xanax, Ativan, and others) that are excellent for treating anxiety and insomnia, can cause a memory loss of the anterograde *type. For example, after taking one of those medications, you can watch a movie or read something, and then a short time later not be able to recall any of the details of the movie or what you read. But that effect is usually transient, and does not continue to be a problem if the medication is taken on a regular basis at therapeutic doses.*

Alcohol is notorious for causing the kind of memory losses you describe. That is usually in the later stages of alcoholism but can occur earlier. From your comments about your husband and family, it does not sound as though you have a problem with alcoholism — but this would be the time to review that possibility in an honest light: Do you drink alcoholic beverages? How much? How frequently? These are questions that you need to review for yourself; ask yourself, are you being entirely honest with yourself? Alcoholism is often overlooked, minimized or denied.

Then there is drug abuse to consider. "Recreational" use of drugs such as marijuana can have a deleterious effect on brain function over time, and some people are much more sensitive and vulnerable to this deterioration than others.

Hopefully you will see a neurologist for a more in-depth examination. You may want to visit a medical center that has more extensive neurological and psychological testing facilities, if one is available in your area.

Good luck, and thanks for writing.

✉✉✉

Incest Survivor

<<I am a incest survivor and I am currently 56 years old. I was recently diagnosed a few months ago with complex PTSD [Post-Traumatic Stress Disorder]. I am seeing a psychiatrist for meds (Celexa, Xanax, and Ambien) and a psychologist for behavior therapy weekly.

My psychiatrist told me I have had PTSD my entire life (abuse started at age 3) and my avoidance-coping mechanisms broke down when I was hospitalized recently for TIA's [Transient Ischemic Attacks — minor strokes] and I had plenty of time to "think."

The meds he has put me on have made me feel much better to the point that I don't want to think about the abuse issues. The docs have encouraged me to consult with lawyers, etc., and I now have a restraining order, since the abuse has still been ongoing. I have been very secretive about it and no one knew. I am very good at avoidance.

My question is: Are the medications starting to work and that is why I am avoiding facing the issue again in therapy or is this a natural symptom of PTSD?

Thank you,
Gloria>>

⊠⊠⊠

Dear Gloria,

Trauma survivors tend to avoid facing the problem because they are unable to deal with it. Once they are successful at working through some of the emotional pain, depression, anxiety, and other

---

symptoms, they are then able to "put it away" or "put it behind" themselves and go on with their lives. That is different from "avoidance" and it is a healthy sign.

The medications you are taking — Celexa (citalopram) for depression; Xanax (alprazolam) for anxiety, and Ambien (zolpidem) for insomnia, are all very effective (but Xanax treats insomnia, too, so you may want to talk to your psychiatrist about whether you actually need both Ambien and Xanax). On the other hand, if the combination is working well for you, without problems or side effects, it may be best to continue on the combination.

You stated that "the abuse is ongoing," so I assume you are not talking about "recovered memories." Recovered Memory Syndrome is a very problematic and questionable psychological diagnosis which often turns out to be spurious. Patients under the care of a psychotherapist, who suddenly recall abuse that occurred in childhood, should be very cautious about accepting those memories as factual. If your memories suddenly arose after you were hospitalized for your TIA's, it is important to evaluate their accuracy extremely carefully.

I cannot advise you about contacting a lawyer. It is not clear what your goal would be; and legal counseling can be very expensive. You would need to be clear in your own mind about what you hoped to accomplish. On the other hand, if you are being physically or sexually abused on an ongoing basis, you may want to consider calling the police and filing charges. Apparently you have already taken some steps in that direction by obtaining a restraining order. However, you – and possibly others – would be safer and more secure if you filed criminal charges and had the perpetrator incarcerated.

Good luck, and thanks for writing.

⊠⊠⊠

<<Thank you for the reply!

I told the lawyers that I could not handle court. They are not happy with my current decision because they felt if anyone could put him away for life, it would be me. I feel that I have enough problems to handle right now dealing with myself.

It was not my desire to involve the legal system; however, my psychologist talked me into a restraining order at the minimum due to my continued contact and my inability to stop the abuse.

My parents are no longer speaking to me. I feel like I am losing my mind and I wonder constantly why I am fighting this. I certainly hope the pain is worth whatever benefits I will get. I am only continuing therapy because I realize now how "messed up" I really am. Hiding the truth for 50 years seems to have caused a lot of damage I was unaware of.

Gloria>>

⊠⊠⊠

Dear Gloria,

Sometimes the cure feels worse than the disease. You need to protect yourself, and it sounds as though you are doing everything you can. Hopefully some day you can forgive your parents for their shortsightedness and narrow view. But remember, you are the greatest source of your own strength and perseverence.

Best of luck to you.

⊠⊠⊠

"My Penis Hurts"

<< In a possible post-divorce custody action, four year old boy makes oral statements more than once without predicate in father's presence, such as:

- "My penis hurts," but cannot describe the hurt, its whys or hows, and there is no physical indication of any injury whatsoever;

- "That tickled my penis" referring to his sensation when traveling over a bump in the road in a motor vehicle;

- Also, child becomes very upset in father's home describing situation where mother's very masculine girl friend painted his toe nails with finger nail polish; nails indeed appeared to have been so polished;

- Child has frequent nightmares and talks of supernatural entities pursuing him in dreams. Child has demonstrated disruptive, noncooperative and assaultive behaviors (relative to peers) in more than one preschool on various occasions; these behaviors were not initially disclosed to child's father who was living elsewhere at time.

Child's father becomes concerned upon learning of behavior problems, returns to town, develops rapport with first school's preschool staff, mother removes child from first school, says it costs too much (although support has increased) and puts him in another school, and problems start again at new preschool. Now child has been referred to local behavior modification program;

child psychologist becomes involved suggests child may be ADD *[Attention Deficit Disorder, sometimes including hyperactivity]*.

It is established that the 4 year old boy's mother was sexually abused, including intercourse, in her home when 6-10 years of age by step father. This sex abuse occurred with at least her own mother's knowledge (boy's grandmother) and acquiescence. Boy's mother is quite intelligent, very successful business woman, in her 30's. Is known to have had a least two sustained "friendships" with very masculine women, but is not overtly so herself, indeed has had heterosexual relationships, but not long term successful ones.

Father fears 4 year old has been sexually abused, or otherwise traumatized and resists possible ADD diagnosis. Father believes child's mother maintains contact with her mother, who is still married to her daughter's perpetrator and has exposed child to this rather bizarre family group, despite divorce decree having "no contact provision" relative to this stepfather. I understand no testing has been done to further ADD suggestion.

Are father's fears justified? If so, what action/intervention would you suggest, since child psychologist isn't buying father's concerns?

Thank you very much for your input.
Robin>>

⊠⊠⊠

Dear Robin,

I am assuming from your comments that you are either the boy's father, or his attorney, or a close friend of the father. Your letter suggests a strong interest in casting the boy's mother in the most negative possible light.

The psychological signs and symptoms you describe of the boy's behavior, comments, and nightmares, may be consistent with sexual abuse — but they are also consistent with those of a child whose divorced parents continue to fight with each other. That may not be uncommon for divorced parents with young children; but it can be psychologically detrimental to the child.

If parents divorce in order to stop fighting and thereby ease tensions for everyone, then divorce can be a "positive" thing. However, when the tension, fighting, and acting out on the part of the parents continues, and the child feels like a tennis ball in play, the destruction to his psyche only intensifies.

(1) The boy should be examined by a medical doctor for any physical signs of abuse. Are there any scratches, marks, or lacerations around his penis or anus? That being said, sexual abuse of sons by their mothers (or other women) is far less common than that perpetrated on daughters by their fathers or male relatives.

(2) The masculinity of the mother's girlfriend is not an issue. If neither the mother, her girlfriends, boyfriends, nor the grandparents are physically abusing the child, then the presentation of the mother's friends is not relevant.

It would seem that a second professional opinion is in order. A child psychiatrist or psychologist should be contacted for a second opinion. The concern about sexual abuse vs. ADD and/or another diagnosis may be sorted out, but the professional should have expertise in those areas.

Most important of all would be ongoing counseling for both parents, and working together with the school staff to sort out the boy's problematic behavior. The parents must find a way to get along for their son's sake. Just the appearance of the parents working together harmoniously with each other and with the school can only have a positive effect on the boy's progress. The parents can go on living their own separate lives and pursuing happiness in their own ways — but for the sake of their child, they need to stop sniping at each other and looking for trouble. Both should be going to the pre-school together to work out an understanding of the boy's problems at school; and both should be seeing a psychologist or family counselor together.

Children can grow up happy and well-adjusted if their parents are "happily" or at least "amicably divorced."

Good luck and thanks for writing.

✉✉✉

Cerebral Hemorrhage

<< Dear Dr. Roth,

Can you recommend a good neuropsychiatrist practising in the Denver,Co, region? Or simply a neurologist who might treat someone with a psychiatric diagnosis?

My daughter suffered a cerebral hemorrhage when she was 9 years old. It was due to the bursting of a congenital venous anomaly in the executive speech center of the brain. Seven months later she was operated on by a doctor (now retired for quite some time) at a world-famous medical center. The surgery went through the left temporal lobe, via a tunnel of dead tissue caused by the bleed, to reach the site and obliterate the tangle of abnormal veins.

My daughter eventually recovered speech (probably because a secondary speech center had developed on the right side of the brain perhaps stimulated at a very early age, possibly prenatal, by the irritation of the venous anomaly). Her behavior following the surgery, however, grew increasingly more difficult throughout her teens. She finished college a year before she was diagnosed as manic-depressive (bipolar I) and later completed a master's degree in teaching English as a foreign language.

However, she has never been consistently compliant with taking medications (the longest period of compliance having been about two years), has been hospitalized several times, and has never found a psychiatrist she both likes and trusts.

Most of the EEG's she has had have shown a normal brain wave, but the one time she was given an EEG with naso-pharyngeal leads, the result was an abnormal brain wave. That was 10 years ago.

She has very long periods of mania and of depression with only a brief interval between them.

I feel that my daughter might be persuaded to see a neurologist; I don't think I'll ever be able to get her to see another psychiatrist voluntarily. Most of those she's seen both in private practise and in clinics have been pretty cold fish. Moreover, there are few psychiatrists in private practise here who are willing to take on new patients with very severe mental illness. And none of them take Medicaid/Medicare patients (understandably because the payment is so little) but I would pay if there were anyone she would see.

My daughter is currently suffering frequent, severe headaches, has been in a manic phase for several months, and has agreed to taking only carbamazapine; but I'm not sure how regularly she takes it. Under court order (Driving While Intoxicated) she is attending an outpatient clinic once every week or two — and getting very little out of it, I think, except for the prescription for carbamazapine. She's now 41 years old—and it's been pretty hellish for much of the last 27 years.

I hope she might have better results with a neurologist or a neuropsychiatrist. (I can't find a listing of a single neuropsychiatrist in the area.)

This is probably a lot more than you ever wanted to read in an email, but I appreciate your attention.

Thank you,

A very worried and sorrow-plagued mother. Lazlo>>

✉✉✉

Dear Lazlo,

You have been dealing with a very difficult situation, and the first thing I want to do is to give you some links to organizations which I feel may help you. One is the National Alliance for the Mentally Ill (N.A.M.I.) which was founded by parents of mentally ill adult children, and can be a great resource for you. The other is the American Neuropsychiatric Association, and from there you may locate a neuropsychiatrist in your area. Here are the links:

National Alliance for the Mentally Ill
http://www.nami.org/

American Neuropsychiatric Association
http://www.neuropsychiatry.com/ANPA/index.html

Another option is to check with your local county mental health department. They often have psychiatrists available for a sliding scale fee. Try to negotiate with your daughter to see "one more" psychiatrist.

You also mentioned that your daughter was ticketed for Driving While Intoxicated, so substance abuse or alcoholism is also in the picture, even though you did not focus on that. Alcoholism is a frequent factor when bipolar patients become manic and reach for something to calm themselves or help them sleep. That, obviously, is very destructive and only serves to make the situation worse. If she has not, or will not consider going to Alcoholics Anonymous, you may want to look into Al-Anon, an organization for family members of those who suffer from alcoholism. Here is a link to their website:

Al-Anon/Alateen Organization
http://www.al-anon.org/

Ultimately, though, your daughter needs to take account of her own life, and decide if taking medication is worse than the hospitalizations — and potential incarceration — that may result from not taking it. It needs to be her decision. She sounds highly intelligent, smart, and competent to assess these factors and make a decision.

Most importantly, I would encourage you to sit back, take a breath, and review the energy you have spent trying to help your daughter. Are you working harder on her problems than she is? Just keep letting her know that you love her, but that you are not going to "rescue" her any more — because the truth is, she is the only one who can rescue herself. You cannot do that if she will not do it. You cannot fail her; and she cannot fail you — only she can fail herself. You have done all that you can.

✉✉✉

<< Dear Dr. Roth,

Thank you for your reply. I have long been a member of NAMI and will definitely look into the other link you sent me. I've been hearing for many years from many sources the advice to pretty much cut loose and let my daughter bottom out. I've been trying to do that, but I fear that in her case the bottom is going to be the end. I wish I knew the statistics on how often that approach works.

Again, thank you. Lazlo>>

✉✉✉

Dear Lazlo,

I do not have the statistics, but you must accept the fact that you cannot save your daughter from herself. That is the most important hurdle for you to leap. If she does not turn herself around, you cannot do it. If your daughter ultimately, God forbid, does herself in, it will be because that is the path she chose. You must have faith, continue to love her, give her the emotional support you always have, and let her live her life as she chooses.

Best of luck to you both.

⊠⊠⊠

<< Dear Dr. Roth,

I'll try to take your advice to heart. Is it possible this illness is harder on me than it is on my daughter?

Thanks again. >>

⊠⊠⊠

Dear Lazlo,

I wouldn't say that — It is hard for you and for her in different ways. But yes, it is very hard on you. You have to take care of yourself. Remember: You cannot help your daughter if you are falling apart over the situation.

Good luck to you and your daughter.

⊠⊠⊠

Alcohol-Related Dementia

<<Dear Dr. Roth: I am a recovering alcoholic. I first got sober about 4 years ago, a couple of months after my children were taken away by the Dept. of Children and Family Services. I had to undergo a psychiatric evaluation which lasted five hours. The previous evening I drank a fifth of vodka. Believe it or not, I passed the evaluation even though I reeked of alcohol. It was deemed that I had alcohol-related dementia, I am narcissistic and histrionic. Eventually I got my children back.

My children again were taken away after my relapse 2 years ago. I drank for three days. I consumed a 12 pack of beer and two fifths of vodka. I again had to take a psych eval (the same one). This time I was sober, but very nervous. Again it was deemed that I suffer from alcohol-related dementia, I am narcissistic and histrionic. It was recently discovered that I am bipolar. I take lithium for this. Now this time the social worker is recommending that my children be put up for adoption.

Could you possibly explain what alcohol-related dementia is? Could you explain what exactly causes the dementia and what part of the brain is damaged? I understand that once you abstain from alcohol it can be reversed to a certain extent.

Is it possible that my dementia continued or was it exacerbated by my relapse. I hold down a job, pay all of my bills, and make my own decisions. I am fully functioning in every capacity and planning to get my Masters degree in 2 years.

Please help me make some sense of this.

Sincerely,
Marina>>

⊠⊠⊠

Dear Marina,

Alcohol-related dementia may refer to two distinct syndromes (clusters of symptoms), one of which is Korsakoff's dementia, the other Wernicke's encephalopathy. Korsakoff's is a memory deficit, usually the inability to lay down longer-term memories. These patients can recall information for a few minutes, but not a few hours or days later. Yet they would still recall earlier, "remote" memories, such as those from childhood, and other years fairly long past.

Wernicke's encephalopathy refers to a difficulty in maneuvering steadily, and a shaking or trembling, often affecting the eyes. Thiamine, also known as vitamin B1, should be given to improve the condition and prevent further deterioration. However, abstaining from alcohol completely is absolutely essential for recovery.

I cannot comment on your diagnosis, as I have not examined you personally. However, if you indeed wrote your letter yourself and have accomplished all of the ongoing tasks and academic achievements you described, it is difficult to conceive of your suffering from dementia. Do see another psychiatrist, possibly a neuropsychiatrist, and/or a psychologist who can repeat the psychological testing to determine your diagnosis with more certainty.

Don't put too much stock in personality testing that shows you to be "this- or that- type." These tests can be very helpful in differentiating between certain diagnoses, such as determining whether someone is severely depressed or actually demented; but in other cases they can do more harm than good. Telling patients that they have a "personality disorder" can affect their self-esteem, or their feelings about themselves and their motivation for recovery.

George Vaillant, a psychiatric researcher, followed over 600 subjects from the 1940's for over 50 years, studying the effect of alcoholism on personality characteristics, and vice-versa. His research revealed how personalities appear to "change" once an alcoholic stops drinking. The deceptiveness and antisocial activity required of an alcoholic — lying about their whereabouts, sometimes stealing or hiding extra money to pay for the addictive substances — affects the way they relate to everyone and everything around them. Once they are clean and sober, their "personality" normalizes, and the antisocial aspects can disappear.

The most important thing for you to do is to keep on with your recovery from alcohol. Find an Alcoholics Anonymous group near you in which you are comfortable and can get the extra support you will need. If you don't feel comfortable among the people in one AA group, try another. There are many around. Check the telephone book for a church or community center that may host AA meetings in your area.

Ask your doctor about Antabuse (disulfiram) which is a medication that helps you to abstain from drinking, because it will cause a sickening response when combined with alcohol. (You must be fairly healthy otherwise, as the response can be severe enough to require an emergency room visit.) Talk about other medications which may help you to abstain from alcohol, such as antidepressants.

Keep going, and good luck to you and to your children. They will always love you best when you are sober.

✉ ✉ ✉

Overly Concerned About Tarantulas

<<Dr Roth —

After several wonderful years on Zyprexa I developed an allergy to it and had to be taken off it. My psychiatrist has put me on 15 mg of Risperdal. I see things in the corner of my eye that aren't there and I am overly concerned about tarantulas (yes, that's right — the hairy spiders). These are new symptoms. I never experienced anything like this while I was on Zyprexa. My only complaint about Zyprexa was weight gain.

Also, on tonight's episode of Ally McBeal they specifically said that Risperdal can be "fatal" to alters *[Alter Ego: See Glossary]* when taken by people with DID *[Dissociative Identity Disorder: See Glossary]* such as myself. Needless to say this was very upsetting. Is there any truth to that or was this just a TV plot line? Why would they specifically refer to Risperdal repeatedly until they finally treated the patient with it against her will causing the "death" of the core (original) personality?

I am going to tell my psychiatrist about the tarantulas and the things in the corner of my eye. I am also made very sleepy by this medicine so I really hope he does not ask me to increase the dosage, but something has to be done. Maybe what I am experiencing is just a temporary side effect.

Any thoughts, advice, etc. would be sincerely appreciated.

Very best regards,
Misha

✉✉✉

Dear Misha,

You are doing the exactly right thing in telling your psychiatrist about the new symptoms you are experiencing (spiders, vision in the corner). There are a dozen or more different medications in the class that includes Zyprexa (olanzapine) and Risperdal (risperidone) that can be effective for your symptoms. There is no reason to stick with Risperdal when it is not working as well as Zyprexa did; or Zyprexa, which caused unacceptable weight gain. Your psychiatrist can offer you trials of other medications which may work as well or even better. Two of the newer ones, Abilify (aripiprazole) and Geodon (ziprasidone), and some of the older ones such as Stelazine (trifluoperazine) and Navane (thiothixene) are not known for causing excessive sedation or weight gain – but there is, as always, a great deal of individual variation in response.

I must report that the TV plot was bunk. Perhaps the actor-patient was convinced that risperidone could "kill" the "alter" personality. I cannot explain why the writers would portray it that way, except that their job is to produce drama. If a patient's "alter ego" represented a psychotic state (which it can be), and they take an anti-psychotic medication (which risperidone is), the patient's mental state could re-integrate — normalize, or come back together — into one baseline personality. Hopefully, there would be no further "splitting" into different "personalities" after that. I suppose you could refer to it as "killing the alter."

However, it is always a shame when a television or movie portrays a medication in such a way as to stigmatize it. Every time I see that — especially with overly dramatized news-magazine types of reports — it makes me sad. People are, in general, very reluctant to take psychiatric medication, and those shows can make it even more difficult.

The fact is that the psychiatric medications are life-saving because they can prevent people from committing suicide. Even patients who are not depressed or suicidal can become frightened enough by auditory and visual hallucinations to become suicidal.

These medications can prevent the need for them to be admitted to psychiatric hospitals over and over again. Risperdal, Zyprexa, and the earlier medications, such as Thorazine or Haldol, treated those symptoms and enabled many people, to regain their sanity and live productive lives.

There are not many medications that can make that dramatic of a statement of fact. Please take a look in the Appendix: History of Thorazine.

Good luck to you, and thanks for writing.

✉✉✉

Time for Yourself?

dear dr. roth:

Hi, I am a high school junior, and I'd like to ask you a few questions. I love psychology and have decided that my career will be in psychiatry. Knowing how strenuous the journey is to go through medical school and then another 4 years for residency, I'd like to ask: did you find it difficult (as busy as you were) to have time for yourself, such as getting married? Family is very important to me, and having to go through another 12 years of studying (after high school) is a bit scary to me, in terms of whether or not I'd have time to start a family before I'm 30. Thanks!
<<LaVerne

⊠⊠⊠

Dear LaVerne,

These are difficult choices to make — there is no question about that. We rarely can make our ideal plans work out exactly as we wish. The answer to your question depends on when you meet "Mr. Right"— or "Dr. Right," as the case may be — before, during or after you have completed your schooling and training.

Getting married is not the biggest problem, as long as you find someone who understands the extra time commitment required of medical schooling and practice. Marriage can help to save money, if you are married and sharing expenses. Having children is a different story. Today, in this present atmosphere of equality & diversity, many medical schools and residency programs make allowances for family planning. You may be able to take some time off your residency to have children, and finish your training later. However, I do not recommend that if you can avoid it.

The best plan is to complete your residency without a lengthy, elective break. It is my opinion that it is better to delay having children, if possible, until after you have completed your residency training. At that point you can look for a flexible work situation which meets your family needs. Consider choosing a medical specialty that allows more flexibility and is more family-friendly. Psychiatry is probably one of the best in that regard. Also, consider working in a group that provides cross-coverage, or an institution that has a generous sick leave/family leave allowance.

Also be sure to take a look at the "Frequently Asked Questions" section of my website for more information about "Psychiatry as a Career."

Good luck, and thanks for writing.

✉✉✉

Bulimia, Epilepsy, Alcoholism and BPD

Dear Dr. Roth:

My 22 year old daughter is about to be discharged after more than 9 months committed to a state mental hospital. She is extremely bulimic (has been purging every day for 5 years) and has been diagnosed with BPD *[Borderline Personality Disorder]*. The bulimia developed in college, out of state, and she was first treated for it at the hospital in her college town, then she came home. The bulimia became so severe, she was arrested for stealing food from the market several times.

All the time she's been at the state hospital there has been no therapy, no treatment except trying every drug imaginable and every combination. The focus was solely on monitoring her weight (currently 87 lbs, 5'5"). Although they are trying to come up with a structured day program, I am not at all optimistic.

Finally, here is my question. When she was 6 yrs old, she began having what seemed like very intense but very brief "panic attacks." An EEG indicated "absent mal" epilepsy as did others in the years that followed. She was on Depakote until she entered high school at which point she adamantly refused to take it (insisting the epilepsy was gone). Her neurologist did another EEG and told her she needed to continue taking Depakote, but when she still insisted on stopping, he said okay, let's try it (without Depakote). She went all through high school without the "panic attacks" or if she had them, she wouldn't admit it. She excelled at swimming and soccer.

During her first hospital commitment several years ago, they put her on Depakote again, and I think she did better but in the years that followed she was taken off it. She began binge drinking and had numerous ER admits for seizures, 4 or 5 were grand mal. (When she returned from the college hospital, she was on Prozac plus Ritalin for ADD *[Attention Deficit Disorder]*.) I understand she is mentally ill but I'm also wondering if epilepsy could be a major contributor — that they produce some intense reactions and she uses food and alcohol as a way to "treat" the feelings they produce.

I am at a loss and trying hard not to lose hope. Thank you for listening, for being willing to accept questions by email. It is so encouraging to see psychiatry and neurology finally coming together.

Maude>>

⊠⊠⊠

Dear Maude,

Epilepsy can manifest itself in unusual ways. "Panic attacks" are not the usual way in which petit mal (or absence seizures) manifest themselves, but if that was diagnosed, then your daughter should take medication for it. It is not clear why she did not want the Depakote — it is known for causing weight gain — but if she had unpleasant side effects, there are other medications which her neurologist may try.

You mentioned several different illnesses, though — bulimia (binge eating) and alcoholism, which makes diagnosis more difficult. Borderline Personality Disorder is kind of a catch-all diagnosis which essentially describes someone who is not psychotic, but cannot pull things together and make their life work well. That diagnosis often applies to individuals who are self-destructive or self-injurious in some way.

Even though your daughter may not be overtly psychotic (out of touch with reality), she may benefit from a small dose of anti-psychotic medication along with her anti-seizure medication. I stress the "small dose" because larger doses of these medications cause side effects, and that makes it less likely that the paitent will continue to take medication. A small dose of an anti-depressant may also be combined with the other medications to help alleviate the need to binge, on both alcohol and food.

You may want to contact a group which can be very helpful for family members of psychiatric patients, regardless of their diagnosis, the National Alliance for the Mentally Ill. Here is their website address:

National Alliance for the Mentally Ill
http://www.NAMI.org

As you said at the end of your letter, you "understand that she is mentally ill," but you are hoping that the epilepsy somehow holds the key to her recovery. Proper medication to treat her impulses is very important, but it is essential that she stops drinking. That is exacerbating all of her illnesses, including epilepsy, as seizures often occur following an alcoholic binge.

Keep up your own spirits, continue to be supportive, but think about accepting your daughter's illnesses. She can get better, but you must begin by accepting her for herself.

Good luck, and thanks for writing.

⊠⊠⊠

Racing Thoughts

<<Dear Dr. Roth,

I know I have a problem I just am not sure what it is and I need your help. I guess I will start from the beginning. I started college when I was 18 and during my first semester I had some sort of breakdown. Well, here is what happened—I was doing very well but I have a huge fear of talking in front of people. Well anyway there was a lot of encouragement in the class from both teacher and students so it helped. The problem started when I began what I call racing thoughts through my head. I would go over and over points that were said good or bad and then it even became delusional to where I thought the teacher had to be plotting something. The more I think about it now I suppose maybe I just couldn't believe I was doing ok in the class.

Anyway I did go to the hospital for 2 weeks and they put me on Risperdal. I think another drug Haldol was used first but it had a lot of side effects. I was really thinking crazy at time. This was the only instance I have ever been delusional. I am now 25. I have been on Zyprexa and Zoloft since and my doctor says that I am a success story for him. The thing is, I only go see him for 10 minutes and I am not completely honest with him because I feel inadequate. He has labled me as "schizoaffective" and says maybe that is not correct — but I am not all together sure he is right because I have a hard time talking to him and telling him everything that is going on. I've wondered whether I am everything from Bipolar, Schizophrenia, and Mania to Avoidant Personality disorder.

Well here is what has been going on since that episode. I have never been delusional like I said — thank God. That was very scary. I do however still suffer from racing thoughts. I have, I think, narrowed the trigger of them down to what I call new situations that occur to me. To explain, I have always been a very quiet person, and to myself, or the introverted type. I had never had any close relationships outside of family until the last two years. I hadn't had any friends that I spent time with and in fact kind of avoided situations where I might have encountered such relationships. It is not that I don't want these relationships — I do — I am just afraid of something but I don't know what and it creates this anxiety in me. While in high school I was afraid to go into stores for some reason.

I spent some time with a psychologist and he really helped me a lot but he moved away. It started out as what seems simple to most people, but for me was very terrifying. I had to go to Burger King and eat. Silly right? Well it got me started anyways. I did that a few times and got used to it and of course I had the racing thoughts along with it. I would do things like rerun an entire conversation back through my head how it should have been done or shouldn't have or what bothered me about it. This is definitely not what I call "back to normal" like before my episode at college.

Well therapy progressed and I came to the conclusion that I should work in a place with people around to overcome my fear of meeting and talking to people. I didn't know how far I would go with this, though. Of course I had all kinds of horrible what-if-this-happens thoughts. Nevertheless I went through with it and got a job at a local amusement park.

Well I was very nervous at first and of course had lots of racing thoughts. I have been there for 8 years now and am the Training Supervisor and am the direct supervisor of 34 employees. Boy, did I change in that respect. The thing is, though, it is a controlled environment and as long as something new doesn't happen to trigger my racing I am ok. I have a lot of friends at work now and over the last 2 years have become very close with several and we go out and to eat a lot and just talk. They are great.

Now I have started a new job working for a large corporation because I finally finished my degree in Business Administration. I am just starting to get in the door however, meaning that I am going to be faced with a lot of challenging situations. I think I will be able to handle this ok but the racing is my biggest problem. What is wrong with me?

Something else that has developed to eliminate these thoughts, I suppose, is that I might "cuss" just to stop this thought process. I get so angry that I might yell out a four-letter word four times in a row and it seem to at least stop this racing for a short moment anyways. The strange thing is this only happens when I am alone or at home. I seem to be able to control it so there must be some hope for me. I just don't know what it is. It just drives me crazy and I feel so ashamed that this is happening to me and I don't know what to do. What is wrong and what can be done?

Ronnie>>

⊠⊠⊠

Dear Ronnie,

My first impression is that you have a tendency to sell yourself very short — you are severely lacking in self-esteem. You have accomplished feats which the average person cannot do — you have succeeded in being promoted to a job with a high level of responsibility supervising many people. That in and of itself shows your tremendous capability. You did this in spite of having an emotional disorder serious enough to require hospitalization and medication.

If that isn't enough, you went on to graduate from college in a highly competitive field of study, and land yourself a good job. So, to begin with, you are well above average in your intelligence, perseverence, and abilities. There is no reason to believe that you will not be successful in your new position, although it sounds like a very challenging one. You have met and conquered such challenges since you were in high school.

With respect to your symptoms, your racing thoughts are suggestive of a bipolar disorder, also known as manic-depressive disorder. You did not mention whether you were on lithium, which was the first and still very effective medication for bipolar disorder. If you have not had a trial of lithium, you may want to talk with your doctor about it. Other medications for bipolar disorder include the anti-seizure medications and the major tranquilizers, or neuroleptics. You are taking Zyprexa (olanzapine), which is a neuroleptic (anti-psychotic) and can be very helpful in bipolar disorder.

The Zoloft (sertraline) which you are taking is an anti-depressant. The more recent development you described — cursing when you are under great stress — is suggestive of a Tourette's syndrome. However, your ability to control it and contain it to times when you are at home dictates against this diagnosis. It is wonderful that your doctor calls you a "success story" because of your personal successes, but that does not mean that you should settle for a medication regimen which leaves you with considerable distress. There is room for improvement in your "inner" level of success, with your symptoms.

When you are under more stress, you may need to increase your dose of medication. You may also benefit from a minor tranquilizer on particularly stressful days. If you have no history of alcoholism or drug abuse, and if those tendencies do not run in your family, then you may benefit from minor tranquilizer medications for anxiety.

You need to discuss all of this with your psychiatrist, who is prescribing your medications. He cannot help you if you are not completely honest with him about your symptoms. You should not try to "protect" his sense that you are "his success story" if you are still having symptoms. If you do not feel that he is doing all that needs to be done, you may want to get a second opinion. You can call a medical center hospital or local mental health agency clinic to get an appointment with another psychiatrist. Be sure he is Board-certified in psychiatry, and is knowledgeable about medication treatments for psychiatric disorders.

Good luck, and thanks for writing.

⊠⊠⊠

Anxiety, Panic, Depression, Depersonalization

<< Dr. Roth,

I have a few questions for you. I am a 37-year-old female. I have been taking imipramine for 10 years. I began taking it after a major depressive episode marked with severe anxiety and panic attacks. I began with 150 mg. a day and finally weaned down to 25 mg. after a period of several years. It took me years to actually recover from this.

There are only two other times I have had what I call a relapse. The first time was in February of 2000, and the second time is now. The first recurrence was caused by the fact that I completely went off of the 25 mg. of imipramine I was taking. A few days went by and I was fine. I wasn't having any of the withdrawal symptoms that I normally had when I missed a dose or tried to stop taking it (nightmares, shakiness, headaches, and general feeling of malaise).

Anyway, I was completely off of the imipramine for I guess about 1-2 wks. All of my symptoms returned with a vengeance (extreme generalized anxiety, panic attacks, and depersonalization — this one is the worst of all). Finally, I knew I was in trouble when the depression came back with terrifying force. I had forgotten how completely debilitating it could be. I began to take my imipramine again at the 25 mg. level. I didn't get better. I went on like this until July of 2000. Why it didn't occur to me that I would need to take more of the medicine than 25 mg., I don't know. My family doctor performed a blood test to check the level of the medicine in my bloodstream. It found none. I went up to 50 and then 75 mg., and then came back to 50, which I stayed on until now. After about 3-4 short weeks, I was back to normal. All of the anxiety gone, no more depersonalization, no depression. It was great.

This brings me to my current problem. About a month or so ago, I began to dream again at night. This is the first sign that I'm about to have some kind of problem relating to my medication. If I ever missed a dose, I had nightmares. Before my first relapse, I dreamed every night. For some reason when I am on this medication, I don't dream at all. That is how I know all is well. I know that sounds weird. Anyway, I knew something was up, but I had not missed a dose nor reduced the dose. I was still taking 50 mg. since July 2000. (I've never been able to get back down to my original 25mg.)

Then a couple of weeks ago I began to experience depersonalization feelings, anxiety and now brief episodes of depression. I cannot explain to you how terrified I am. There are no words. I don't know what has brought this on. My question is, could I become immune to imipramine after taking it for so long? I'm terrified of this. I've tried many of the "new generation" antidepressants. They don't help me like imipramine. Could it be extreme stress that would trigger a change in brain chemistry?

I have a sick mother and I am her only caregiver. She was diagnosed this year with a minor stroke. I have been on a whirlwind ever since. She has many hours of therapy each week. I've been on the net looking up information concerning this condition. She also has a heart condition. My life consists of working as a stock clerk part-time, managing my mother's doctor appointments, and therapy appointments, and keeping all of the medical bills and insurance papers organized.

I have a most wonderful, helpful, and understanding husband. So I did have some help. Anyway, I have gone up to 75 mg. I've been there for about 3 weeks now. My symptoms are bearable, but extremely scary. They are in no way full-blown. I'm still working. What could have caused my body to stop responding to the dose I was on? And why is it not responding to the 75 mg? I'm due for another blood level to see what the level is now. My family doctor is just not educated enough in this area. I need advice from a specialist. I need help now. I cannot afford another episode. I'm not there yet, but if the medication does not begin to do its job, that's where I'm headed. Please respond as quickly as you can. I'm sorry this was so long, but I wanted to give you all of the facts.

Thanks,

Margaret in South Dakota>>

☒☒☒

Dear Margaret,

Often when people go off of their medication and relapse, they require a larger dose to get re-stabilized. Imipramine is an old standard antidepressant, and a very good medication. But as you said, you originally started out taking 150 mg. per day. Once your depression and other symptoms were well under control, it was possible to reduce the dose to a much lower "maintenance" dose. That is very common.

There are other medical conditions which respond the same way, even though they are completely different conditions. For example, if you have a bronchial (upper respiratory) infection, your doctor may start you on a double dose of antibiotics on the first day, to build up the blood level of medication quickly. People with diabetes may require a higher dose of insulin when their blood sugar registers a higher level than at other times. Many disease conditions require such dosing adjustments.

The "dreaming" episodes which seems to herald a relapse for you, are probably due to the depressive symptoms interfering with your sleep pattern (depression is notorious for disturbing one's sleep). Everyone spends time in the "REM" (Rapid Eye Movement) sleep stage during which we experience dreaming. That occurs just prior to awakening—and that stage seems to help drive us back down into the deeper stages of sleep. When you are relapsing toward depression, you are not sleeping as deeply. You awaken more easily, and you are tending to recall your dreams more readily than when you are not depressed, and sleeping more deeply.

You must recognize and be prepared for a possible relapse of depression from time to time. You are actually fortunate in a way, that your sleep pattern begins to change before you get seriously ill—that gives you the opportunity to nip it in the bud, so to speak, with an immediate return to higher doses. Others who suffer from depression do not have such a clear sign, or prodrome. Also be aware that depression tends to recur when one is under more stress. That may be increased by your mother's illness.

Keep in mind that a higher dose of medication is needed initially to "get on top of" your symptoms. Then, when you are once again in full remission, you will probably be able to gradually, with your doctor's supervision, reduce the dose back to a maintenance dose, such as the 25-50 mg. you used to take. You may not be able to get back that low, but stay on the dose that works for you. There is nothing wrong with taking a higher dose, especially since you have had such good results from the imipramine.

With respect to your question about the possibility of becoming "immune" to imipramine after taking it for so long—yes, something like that is possible. I do not think "immune" is the right term, though—the medication still helps, but you need higher doses to achieve the same level of remission and stabilization. It is possible that, rather than the medication failing to work, or failing to work as well anymore, your relapses are somewhat more intense than they were in the past. Moreover, our bodies and systems change over time, and that may dictate the need for a different dose, or even a different medication.

It is very important that you find a psychiatrist to work with your medications. He can follow your progress while adjusting the dosages, and may try some of the newer antidepressants which are coming out on the market all the time. He may even try some medications in combination, which would help the imipramine work once again at a lower dose. For example, adding a minor tranquilizer to a low dose of imipramine might allow you to maintain a stable mood and alleviate your anxiety and panic attacks. Psychiatrists are more familiar with prescribing combinations such as these, so you should definitely ask your family doctor for a referral.

Good luck, and thanks for writing.

✉✉✉

Part II.

Medications for...

Depression, anxiety, mood swings, hyperactivity, and even psychosis, can all be the result of other conditions. Certain medical illnesses, such as high- or low-thyroid production, or side effects from medications such as steroids, high blood pressure or acne medication, can produce significant clinical changes in a person's mental functioning. It is very important that a thorough physical exam be conducted by an internal medicine or family practice physician, or a pediatrician, before making a diagnosis and prescribing psychiatric medications.

Anxiety

The most effective anti-anxiety medications, a class of drugs called benzodiazepines, can also be helpful for sleep disorders, muscle relaxation, panic attacks, and some obsessive-compulsive symptoms. This medication is also prescribed to alleviate alcohol withdrawal; and for muscle spasms or muscle strain.

Benzodiazepines are often referred to as "addictive" medication; but for the vast majority of people who take them, that is not the case[3]. They can be safely used on a long-term basis to treat chronic disabling anxiety, panic attacks, and sleep disorders; or in the short-term for situational anxiety, performance anxiety ("stage fright") or the sleep disturbance that accompanies depression and stress. There are no long-term ill effects such as the kind of organ system damage seen with chronic excessive alcohol use, tobacco use, illegal or prescription drug abuse, unless those substances are combined with benzodiazepines.

The recommended dose range may be continued indefinitely, however, even for years, in patients who have chronic severe anxiety disorders, chronic insomnia, or recurrent panic attacks, without any identifiable ill effects. Some patients may adjust their dose from time to time, depending on the amount of stress that is occurring; but for the most part, patients will stay within their initially prescribed dose range.

There are patients who will overuse benzodiazepines. That is usually apparent early in treatment, and the prescription should be tapered and discontinued. On the other hand, if a minimal dose is given at first, and the patient states that he has gotten partial relief but not adequate relief, then a higher dose may be needed. Doses need to be adjusted for the severity of the illness. As long as patients are not excessively drowsy or impaired in any way; or

---

[3] Schatzberg AF, Nemeroff CB, Editors. The American Psychiatric Publishing Textbook of Psychopharmacology, May, 2009. p. 379.

requesting early refills frequently; or claiming that their supply of medication has been "left on the bus" or "stolen" time and time again, there is no reason to assume that they are abusing, misusing or selling their supply of medication.

Patients who require daily chronic anti-anxiety medication should not be considered addicted as long as they are staying within the recommended dose range prescribed by their physician. A person's overall functioning as a result of taking the medication, compared with not taking it, needs to be considered.

Some of the benzodiazepines include:

Brand Name	Generic Name
Librium[4]	chlordiazepoxide
Valium	diazepam
Xanax	alprazolam
Ativan	lorazepam
Klonopin	clonazepam
Halcion	triazolam
Versed	midazolam
Restoril	temazepam
Dalmane	flurazepam
Serax	oxazepam
Tranxene	clorazepate

Buspirone: Anti-anxiety medication which is considered less problematic than the benzodiazepines listed. It is popular for treating patients who have been problem drinkers (alcoholics) or drug abusers, or who have abused or over-used benzodiazepines in the past.

Antihistamines such as Benadryl (diphenhydramine) may benefit an anxious person due to their slightly sedating or drowsying side effect.

Propranolol is a medication prescribed for high blood pressure, palpitations (heart "racing"), or sweating, and can be very

---

[4] Not to be confused with *LITHIUM*, a medication for bipolar disorders.

useful for relieving the temporary anxiety of performing in public ("stage fright").

Clonidine[5] is a medication prescribed for high blood pressure, and is also helpful in opiate (e.g. heroin) detoxification. It can be helpful for anxiety in patients who cannot take benzodiazepines.

Attention Deficit Disorder or Hyperactivity

ADD (Attention Deficit Disorder) and ADHD (Attention Deficit Disorder with Hyperactivity) are treated with stimulant medications, but others may also help. Ritalin, which is the brand name for methylphenidate, and Cylert, or pemoline, are central nervous system stimulants. That means that they activate nerve cells in the brain. A stimulant has a "paradoxical" effect in hyperactive youngsters — that is, it has the opposite effect from what is expected. Instead of activating the child even more, it calms him down and helps him to focus more easily.

It is thought that the stimulant medications stimulate the *inhibitory* neurons in the brain. Inhibitory neurons are nerve cells that *reduce* activity. For example, when someone is listening to music, inhibitory nerve cells actively "screen out" other sounds that are coming in, such as street noises or background conversations. The person *hears* the background street noises and conversations, but he is not *listening* to them—not processing them as information, and probably could not tell you what he heard besides the music.

When methylphenidate and pemoline stimulate the inhibitory nerve cells, it helps hyperactive children to calm down and focus on the task at hand. Otherwise, they may be distracted by every little sight or sound in the area. It may be helpful to consider stimulant medication as similar to the brakes on a car: it takes energy (stimulation) to apply the brakes, which slow the car down.

---

[5] Not to be confused with *clonazepam* (Klonopin), a benzodiazepine.

Stimulant medication *activates the brakes* and slows the child down, allowing him to focus on the task.

Depression

Antidepressants have been lifesavers for literally millions of people who suffer from depression. Psychiatry has over a fifty-year history with antidepressant medication [see "The History of Antidepressants" in Appendix A]. Antidepressants are extremely effective, safe when taken in recommended doses, and have tolerable side effects for most people; that is, the side effects are far more tolerable than the untreated depression.

One of the greatest rewards in psychiatry is to hear a patient say, "You know, I didn't want to take any medication ... But now that I have, I realize I've been depressed all my life ... Now for the first time, I know what it feels like *not* to be depressed." Antidepressants can significantly improve one's quality of life.

The original antidepressants, tricyclics (TCA's) and mono-amine-oxidase inhibitors (MAOI's), are very effective, but can be dangerous in overdose—and with depressed patients, the potential for overdose is always a prominent concern. The more common side effects, dry mouth or constipation, are fairly well tolerated. The newer antidepressants such as the selective serotonin reuptake inhibitors (SSRI's) are just as effective, but less toxic in overdose. Most patients are begun on SSRI's initially now—but if these prove less than adequate to treat the depression, the psychiatrist should not hesitate to return to the old standards for relief.

Hyperactivity (also see Attention Deficit Disorder)

Hyperactivity can also occur without an Attention Deficit. A person may exhibit high energy and excessive movement, while still paying attention and absorbing the information they need to absorb. Some examples of this are people who swing their foot continually while seated; or tap their pencil or fingers constantly when listening to something.) Medication would not be prescribed for this condition (but sedatives may be required for the person sitting next to them in class).

Mood swings

Lithium[6] is a simple element found in nature, and is still the number-one drug of choice for Bipolar Disorder, or Manic-Depressive Illness [see "The History of Lithium" in Appendix A]. Lithium has been correlated with a reduction in suicidal behavior in bipolar and depressed patients. It is an excellent choice to add to an antidepressant for patients with recurring severe depression, even without elevated mood swings.

Other medications shown to be effective with bipolar disorder include the anti-seizure medications: Tegretol (carbamazepine), Depakote (valproic acid), Neurontin (gabapentin), and Lamictal (lamotrigene). Minor tranquilizers (sedative or anti-anxiety medications) and major tranquilizers (neuroleptic or anti-psychotic medications) may be needed. These may or may not have to be continued once the patient is well-stabilized.

Antidepressants should be used with caution in the depressed phase of manic-depressive illness, as they have been known to trigger a "switch" into a manic phase. For that reason, it is helpful to use an anti-manic medication in combination with antidepressant medication for the depressed phase of bipolar disorder. As the mood stabilizes, one or both medications may be reduced and discontinued. However, it is often necessary to remain on one or more medications in lower "maintenance" doses, to avoid a relapse.

---

[6] Not to be confused with *LIBRIUM*, the brand name for chlordiazepoxide — See Anxiety.

Personality Disorders

Personality Disorders are developed over many years, and often require lengthy periods of psychotherapy to have an impact. [See *Part III - Glossary of Terms and Disorders* for more discussion on Personality Disorders.] There is no specific medication that will change a person's personality, but medication can help the same symptoms of depression or anxiety as in others.

Some personality disorders are so severe that they appear to mimic the psychotic disorders [see *Multiple Personality Disorder* and *Borderline Personality Disorder* in the Glossary]. Those persons may benefit from low doses of anti-psychotic medication, in addition to antidepressants for depression, or any other symptoms that require treatment.

One caveat is that a psychotic person may *appear* to have a personality disorder, as a result of his disturbed thinking and behavior. It is important that symptoms of a major mood disorder or anxiety are treated before making a diagnosis of personality disorder, which requires an entirely different approach.

Psychosis

Prior to the 1950's, Thorazine (chlorpromazine) was prescribed to help patients get to sleep. As a "sleeper" it was not ideal, as it took a very long time for the body to metabolize and eliminate from storage, often leaving a "hangover" effect. However, when used on psychotic patients, it was discovered to the delight and amazement of the medical staff that it also improved psychotic thought processes [see "The History of Thorazine" in Appendix A]. When that effect was repeated, and Thorazine use became widespread, the mental institutions and asylums of this country emptied out by fully two-thirds. The per-capita census of hospitalized mental patients has never gone back up since that time.

In the 1960's, the Mental Health Bar of the American Bar Association lobbied for laws to release mental patients based on their "rights" — for example, the right to refuse treatment, regardless of psychotic symptoms. Mentally ill individuals could only be hospitalized, or treated with medication against their will, if they were brought before a judge who determined that they were dangerous to themselves or others (suicidal or homicidal). The mental hospital population diminished even more after that legal activism, referred to as "deinstitutionalization".

Unfortunately, many of the psychiatric patients previously committed to hospitals are now sleeping in streets and doorways, under bridges and on park benches. That is why psychiatrists and lawyers hold a respectful professional disdain for each other. The rest of the world holds disdain for both professions, as in, "The stereotyped psychiatrist 'puts people away against their will,' while the lawyer fights to obtain the release of 'psychotic homicidal maniacs' into a defenseless society." Of course, neither stereotype is accurate (except for the lawyer part).

In the decades since, there have been many new antipsychotic medications developed to improve upon Thorazine's range of action and side effect profile. Antipsychotic medications are also known as *neuroleptics* (from the Greek meaning, "to take hold of the nerves") or *major tranquilizers* (as opposed to the *benzodiazepines*, which are classed as *minor tranquilizers*).

Antipsychotic medication is prescribed for such psychotic symptoms as auditory hallucinations (hearing non-existent voices or sounds), visual hallucinations (seeing non-existent sights); paranoid or other delusional thoughts that have no rational basis in reality; or fragmented thought processes.

Psychotic symptoms can occur in combination with other psychiatric conditions, and often a combination of medication is required. For example, paranoia and auditory hallucinations can occur with depression (particularly common in elderly depressed patients); or as a result of illicit drug use, such as LSD, cocaine, marijuana, and amphetamines; or along with visual hallucinations such as in alcohol psychosis, alcohol withdrawal, or delerium tremens (DT's). In all of these cases, neuroleptics may be used, and may be combined with other drugs such as benzodiazepines or antidepressants.

Antipsychotic medications tend to be very safe, and the range of useful dosing is very broad. For example, early patients were treated with Thorazine in doses ranging from 50 mg. to 2,000 mg. daily. Seroquel can be effective in 25 to 800 mg. daily. The mega-dosing attests to their high level of safety.

Older *"Typical"* Antipsychotics		Newer *"Atypical"* Antipsychotics	
Brand name	*Generic name*	*Brand name*	*Generic name*
Thorazine	*chlorpromazine*	Abilify	*aripiprazole*
Prolixin	*fluphenazine*	Zyprexa	*olanzapine*
Haldol	*haloperidol*	Risperdal	*risperidone*
Stelazine	*trifluoperazine*	Clozaril	*clozapine*
Loxitane	*loxapine*	Geodon	*ziprasidone*
Moban	*molindone*	Seroquel	*quetiapine*
Navane	*thiothixene*	Invega	*paliperidone*
Trilafon	*perphenazine*	Serdolect	*sertindole**
Mellaril	*thioridazine*	Solian	*amisulpride**

*Not approved for use in the U. S.

Part III.

Glossary
of
Terms & Disorders

Particularly annoying in psychiatry is the tendency to re-name mental diseases and disorders from time to time. The Diagnostic and Statistic Manual (DSM) has gone through nearly half a dozen editions, and some disorders have been renamed that many times. For example, Manic-Depressive illness has morphed into Bipolar Affective Disorder; Multiple Personality Disorder has been reintroduced as Dissociative Identity Disorder. Now there is an entity called Anancastic Personality Disorder, which is an old – or a new term, depending on what you read – for Obsessive-Compulsive Personality Disorder. In any case, this section may be helpful in identifying terms for the Reader. Old and new terms will be included where applicable.

ADD or ADHD: Attention Deficit Disorder or Attention Deficit and Hyperactivity Disorder, describes a person, usually a child, who has difficulty focusing, sleeping or resting, concentrating, reading, or — in the case of hyperactivity — remaining quiet or sedentary for any length of time. Contrary to previous thought, residual symptoms of this disorder often continue into adulthood.

Addiction: A craving for something in spite of harmful or unpleasant consequences; constant thinking about and planning for the next opportunity to indulge in the activity; a compulsion to indulge against one's own conscious will to stop. Addiction is highly individual: A cocaine addict or marijuana smoker may have no taste for alcohol, and vice-versa (also see *Alcoholism*). Benzodiazepines such as Valium or Xanax are rarely addictive.

Affective: Pronounced *AFF*-fective (emphasis on the first syllable), refers to emotions or feelings. An *Affective Disorder* is a mood disorder, either depressed, manic, or a combination of mood swings from one to the other (see *Bipolar Disorder.*)

Agoraphobia: Literally, "fear of the marketplace." People with agoraphobia tend to avoid crowds, and may experience panic attacks (see definition). These frequently occur when the person feels "trapped" in a place from which there is no easy exit, such as in a grocery line. Some who suffer from agoraphobia stay at home more and more; and in extreme cases, it may be years since they have ventured outside.

Alcoholism: This is a term that is defined differently by many different criteria. How much is too much? How often is too often? There is a tendency to define alcoholism by the amount of alcohol and the frequency with which it is consumed. However, those parameters are highly debateable. The only clear definition of an alcoholic is one whose drinking interferes with his health, productivity, work, relationships, or involvement with the law.

Alter Ego: "Other self" usually referring to the different "personalities" in persons who suffer from Multiple Personality Disorder (more recently re-named Dissociative Identify Disorder). Alter ego in non-psychiatric circles can be a reference to the different "sides" to someone's personality, such as, "Drinking brings out the dark side of his personality..."

Antisocial Personality Disorder: The antisocial personality is characterized by a general lack of concern for the rights of others. Antisocial persons feel *entitled* to have whatever they are successful in obtaining, and justify breaking the law to do so. Antisocial acts are often justified by attributing blame to the victims themselves. For example, a gang-banger feels justified in beating or robbing someone who has crossed into "his" territory—the victim "deserved" the beating because he entered the gang-banger's territory. A used car salesman may feel justified in deliberately exaggerating a car's road-worthiness—he believes the customer "deserved" to be cheated because of his ignorance about cars and his foolishness in trusting a used-car salesman! (I was actually told this by a former used-car salesman who went to prison for falsifying loan applications.)

Antisocial individuals can also act "within" the law (I refer to these as "Socialized Antisocial Personalities"). They will ignore the rights of others to get what they want, as long as those rights are *not specifically protected by law* or *inconsistently enforced*. For example, an employer who makes sexual advances toward a subordinate who would be fearful of losing her job if she refused, is an example of a "socialized" antisocial personality. The employer does not have to hold his employee at gunpoint, or even verbalize a specific threat—the "silent threat" of losing her job is a "socialized" way of forcing her to acquiesce. (Sexual harassment remains problematic in society in spite of state and federal laws passed in the 1990's and later, since there are usually no witnesses, and victims are reluctant to come forward with charges).

Anxiety: A state of worry or fearfulness for reasons that may or may not be identifiable, rational or based in reality.

Avoidant Personality Disorder: These individuals tend to be shy and lack self-confidence, to a disabling degree. Fear of rejection and an easily wounded sense of self-esteem foster a tendency to avoid people and situations where this may occur, such as not pursuing available opportunities for job advancement.

Borderline Personality Disorder: BPD is a large tent under which many other diagnoses, including other Personality Disorders, are included. Individuals with BPD suffer with chronic, low-grade depression and unfocused anger. They often have poor impulse control, as well as difficulty developing stable relationships. BPD covers a spectrum from "high-functioning" to "low-functioning" individuals. They suffer from the following symptoms, to a greater or lesser degree:

- Substance abuse: Alcoholism and/or drug abuse.
- Multiple intense relationships or short-lived marriages.
- Repeated relationships with abusive partners.
- Frequent suicidal thoughts, gestures or attempts.
- Sexual promiscuity, with or without protection from disease or pregnancy.
- Self-mutilation by such means as extensive body-piercing or tattooing (especially on the face, neck or genitals);
- Self-injurious behavior such as cutting or burning oneself, not necessarily suicidal, but as a means of relieving anxiety.

- Dangerous acting out, such as reckless driving or driving while intoxicated.
- Antisocial behavior.

When under severe stress, people with BPD may experience psychotic symptoms: they may hear voices or have paranoid or other delusions. Small doses of anti-psychotic medication may be helpful at those times. Unlike schizophrenia, in which those symptoms are more chronic, anti-psychotic medication may be discontinued when the BPD patient is no longer under stress.

Bipolar Disorder (Bipolar Affective Disorder): Originally known as "Manic-Depressive Illness", signs and symptoms include excessive mood swings (beyond a normal range), or moods changing more rapidly than normal, or accelerating into psychotic thinking. Periods of high energy, excessive activity and little need for sleep can slide into a severe depression, wherein the patient may stay in bed for days or have suicidal thoughts, with no clear precipitating cause. Psychotic symptoms such as hearing voices, seeing visions, or feeling paranoid can occur in some bipolar patients, and may initially suggest a diagnosis of schizophrenia. Grandiose delusions are not uncommon, such as thinking one is wealthy, famous, or has special powers. Unrestrained shopping sprees due to the delusion of wealth can lead to legal troubles.

Dependent Personality Disorder: Individuals who are diagnosed with Dependent PD tend to lack confidence in their own decision-making ability. They seem to be more in need of assistance than their level of physical and mental competence would suggest. These individuals rely too heavily on a supporter or support system, and are unable — but often accused of being unwilling — to take on an appropriate level of responsibility for themselves.

Depersonalization: a feeling of "detachment" from oneself, as though one is standing outside of oneself, like an observer.

Depression: A feeling of sadness or low mood that can be a normal response to an unhappy or unpleasant situation. *Major Depression* is an abnormal condition that may manifest itself without any apparent cause. It can be accompanied by *vegetative symptoms*, such as sleep disturbance, crying spells, loss of appetite or significant increase in appetite; loss of interest in normally enjoyable activities; fatigue or lack of energy; or other symptoms such as difficulty concentrating; agitation and irritability; and pervasive thoughts of death or suicide.

Depressive Personality Disorder: There is some debate as to whether this is a variant of, or the same as, **Dysthymic Disorder**. This diagnosis is descriptive of folks who just seem unhappy most of the time. They find little joy in anything, but their lackluster feelings about life do not reach the magnitude for a diagnosis of depression. They go about their business, working, marrying, raising children, but do not express the kind of joy normally articulated during "good times," but rather focus on the negative. They can be brooding, given to worry, pessimistic.

Dissociative Identity Disorder: This diagnosis includes Multiple Personality Disorder [which is considered separately in this section] as well as other related "dissociative" conditions: "Psychogenic amnesia," is a condition wherein the person cannot recall very significant memories. In a "Psychogenic fugue" state, an individual travels some considerable distance from their normal location, sometimes into completely unfamiliar territory, without recalling how they got there or how much time elapsed.

Dysthymic Disorder: A low-grade depression that is relatively chronic. Symptoms of depression tend to be more persistent but not as disabling as in Major Depression. There is some debate as to whether **Depressive Personality Disorder** is a variant of, or the same as Dysthymic Disorder.

Epilepsy: Epileptic seizures, historically called "fits" occur when electrical impulses in the brain are triggered involuntarily and send messages that affect the person's movement and consciousness.

- *Gran mal* seizures usually begin on one side of the body, causing large jerking tremors, and travel down that side of the body to the foot. The patient rarely has any recollection of the seizure.

- *Petit mal* seizures are also called *Absence seizures*, and typically occur in school-age children. During the seizure, The child appears as if he is daydreaming. Rapid blinking often accompanies this type of seizure.

- *Temporal Lobe* or *Partial Complex* seizures can have a variety of presentations. Classically, the patient will appear as though he is concentrating on doing some kind of activity such as picking something off his clothing.

Histrionic Personality Disorder: These individuals are excessively emotional and overly dramatic. They seek attention from those around them and thrive on being the center of attention.

Mania: An abnormally high-energy state, or state of irritability, which can include loss or little need for sleep, and poor impulse control and judgment.
Manic-Depressive Disorder: See Bipolar Disorder.

Masochistic Personality Disorder: (Also see Sadistic/ Sadomasochistic Personality Disorder) Sadomasochism is a form of sexual deviation in which the participants inflict or submit to painful or humiliating verbal or physical assault. Activities that would be highly aversive to the majority of individuals are experienced as pleasurable and erotic to the sadomasochistic partners. Sometimes the partners trade places, alternating at playing the sadistic role (inflicting pain or humiliation), and then playing the masochistic role (submitting to the pain or humiliation).

Multiple Personality Disorder: Also called "Dissociative Identity Disorder (covered separately in this section), MPD is more of a major psychiatric disorder—more severe than a simple "personality disorder." This psychiatric disturbance is one in which the patient exhibits different (multiple) *personas*, or *alter egos*, rather than a dysfunction of their true personality.

MPD may be related to schizophrenia—in both, a psychotic break with reality is manifested. Different needs, desires, and (often traumatic) incidents the individual has experienced will "compartmentalize" themselves into separate "personalities."

For example, a woman who was sexually molested as a child may suddenly begin to dress provocatively and frequent less-than-savory establishments late at night. A lapse into an entirely different "personality" that exhibits characteristics completely alien to the "real" self, would represent a fracture in the integrity of the woman's mental functioning. Other needs and desires might follow with yet more "personalities." For example, the need for the protective love and nurturance that was absent from the individual's childhood may develop into a "child" personality, with regressive behavior and a child-like voice. Patients with MPD often require antipsychotic medication along with psychotherapy treatment.

Narcissistic Personality Disorder: "Narcissus" is a mythical figure who fell in love with his own reflection in a pond, fell in and drowned. Those who exhibit NPD have an exaggerated sense of self-importance. They thrive on admiration and feel entitled to it. However, beneath this outward air of superiority is a fragile self-esteem that crumbles or explodes when faced with constructive criticism or reproach.

Obsessive-Compulsive Disorder: "OCD" Refers to a combination of feelings that include obsessing over persistent unwanted thoughts, fears or anxieties; and a compulsion to act on these thoughts in a repetitious manner. A person is diagnosed with *OCD* if he has become significantly disabled by the symptoms. These individuals may require medication and psychotherapy, along with behavior therapy to obtain relief. [See also *Obsessive-Compulsive Personality*].

Obsessive-Compulsive Personality Disorder: Unlike the obsessive-compulsive "types" we all know who are very attentive to detail (sometimes annoyingly so), but stay on task, complete it in a timely manner, and tend to be highly productive, the Obsessive-Compulsive Personality *Disorder* is diagnosed when the attention of the individual spirals into endless focus on smaller and smaller aspects of the details, to the detriment of the project. They are overly focused on rules, regulations and order, so much so that they may have trouble completing a task, or accepting another's task as complete. The individual with OCPD may never feel that a task is sufficiently perfected or completed to their satisfaction.

Palpitations: The feeling that the heart is racing, beating too strongly, or beating irregularly. See *Panic Attack.*

Panic Attack: A sudden feeling of "impending doom." This is often described as feeling that one is about to die. The heart may start racing (palpitations) and sweating may occur, accompanied by a strong need to flee the area. Panic attacks often result in Emergency Room visits that result in the inability to find any physical etiology (cause) for the symptoms. They are diagnosed by the description of the symptoms and the place where they occurred, such as the feeling of "entrapment" in a grocery store line.

Paranoia: A delusional state wherein a person believes that people are interacting with them when there is no basis in reality for such belief. A paranoid individual may believe that people are plotting against him; talking about him; following him; signaling him; laughing at him; or being unfaithful to him. There are instances where these conditions do exist, in reality, so it is important to get adequate background information before making this diagnosis.

Paranoid Personality Disorder: These individuals are suspicious and distrustful by nature. Their concerns do not reach delusional proportions, such as in Paranoid Schizophrenia. But the diagnosis of Paranoid PD is made when the symptoms have begun interfering with normal relationships. For example, a husband who is distrustful of his wife attending a book club every week, even though he has no evidence to believe she is acting out in any improper manner, may be diagnosed with Paranoid PD.

Passive-Aggressive Personality Disorder: Passive-Aggressive PD is found in those who try to control situations by *inaction*. For example, they fail to act when action on their part is required, needed or helpful. They impede progress and cause difficulties for others by deliberately *not* acting. Passive-Aggressive individuals will do what is expected of them, but perhaps too slowly; or intentionally shoddily.

The comedian, Bill Cosby, had a classic routine about his wife's request that he make breakfast for the kids. He was happy to comply. The breakfast consisted of chocolate cake. His wife never asked him to make breakfast again. That's passive-aggressive.

Personality Disorder (PD): "Personality" refers to the style in which an individual interacts with others and manages his own needs and desires. "Disorder" refers to those personality characteristics which impede a person's ability to function smoothly or normally in society. Individuals with PD have more difficulty managing the many stressors, trials and tribulations, that life presents. PD develops over many years, but the origins in childhood can often be seen in retrospect.

   PD generally requires intensive psychotherapy to change; but to be successful, the individuals must recognize their contribution to their own problems and suspend the temptation to attribute blame to others. "How many psychiatrists does it take to change a lightbulb? Only one—but the lightbulb must want to change." This joke, painful in its truthfulness, personifies the individual with PD.

   Medication cannot cure PD, but it can help some of the symptoms, such as a depressed mood. Individuals with PD can get depressed just as others do, and this condition impairs their ability to assess themselves objectively and be successful in so many aspects of their lives. Some examples of Personality Disorders include the following (and further definitions are found under the individual disorders):

>Antisocial Personality Disorder
>Avoidant Personality Disorder
>Borderline Personality Disorder
>Dependent Personality Disorder
>Depressive Personality Disorder
>Histrionic Personality Disorder

Multiple Personality Disorder[7]
Masochistic Personality Disorder[8]
Narcissistic Personality Disorder
Obsessive-Compulsive Personality Disorder[9]
Paranoid Personality Disorder
Passive-Aggressive Personality Disorder
Sadistic/Sadomasochistic Personality Disorder
Schizoid Personality Disorder
Schizotypal Personality Disorder

Pharmacology: the study of medications and how they work in the body (See also Psychopharmacology and Psychotropic).

Post-Traumatic Stress Disorder: "PTSD" is a condition that occurs following a severely stressful situation, usually when one's life has been endangered, or as a result of watching someone else being severely traumatized. PTSD is seen in victims of earthquakes, flood, or other such disasters; major automobile accidents with severe injury or death of others; rape; combat; and terrorist attacks. The victims will "re-live" the events and begin to avoid anything that reminds them of it (such as water, in the case of a flood; riding in an automobile, in the case of an accident; intimacy, in the case of a rape; and so forth). PTSD requires intensive therapy for symptoms such as paranoia, depression, and sleep disturbance; and can lead to drug or alcohol abuse.

Psychiatrist: A medical doctor (M. D.) who has completed college, medical school, and a training program (residency) in Psychiatry. The psychiatric residency training program usually includes a year of Internal Medicine and Neurology, and three years of psychiatric

---

[7] Now known as "Dissociative Identity Disorder."
[8] Also see "Sadistic/Sadomasochistic Personality Disorder."
[9] Obsolete term was "Anancastic" Personality Disorder.

training. A psychiatrist can diagnose mental and physical disorders, and treat them with *medication* when necessary, and *psychotherapy*.

Psychologist: A non-medical practitioner[10] who has usually completed his Bachelors Degree, Masters Degree, and Doctorate in Philosophy (Ph. D.) in the area of Psychology. A psychologist can diagnose mental disorders, conduct a vast array of psychological testing, and treat mental disorders with psychotherapy, often using a variety of techniques, including psychoanalysis, hypnosis, and behavior modification.

Psychopharmacology: the study of medications used in psychiatry, including major and minor tranquilizers, antipsychotic and anti-depressant medications. "Major tranquilizer" and "antipsychotic" are interchangeable terms. "Minor tranquilizer" refers to anti-anxiety medications or sedatives, which can also be useful adjuncts in psychotic conditions. The term "mood stabilizer" can refer to an antidepressant or a medication for manic-depressive (bipolar) patients who suffer from mood swings.

Psychotherapist: A psychiatrist, clinical psychologist, registered nurse practitioner, clinical social worker, or anyone else trained in psychotherapeutic technique, licensed or certified by a state licensing body.

Psychotherapy: Helping to unravel a patient's disturbed thoughts and emotions by listening, asking questions and giving feedback. Psychotherapy can take many forms, including psychoanalysis, behavior modification, relaxation and self-hypnosis.

Psychotropic: Refers to medications that are used in psychiatry.

---

[10] Psychologists have been given limited prescribing privileges for psychotropic medication in New Mexico and Louisiana.

Sadistic / Sadomasochistic Personality Disorder: (Also see Masochistic Personality Disorder). Sadism is the "cruelty" branch of sadomasochism. Sadistic individuals get pleasure, often sexual, from inflicting great pain or humiliation on another person.

Schizoid Personaltiy Disorder: These individuals generally function normally at work and in society; but they are disinterested in social relationships, preferring solitary activities, and showing minimal emotionality.

Schizotypal Personality Disorder: These individuals have significantly odd ideas, beliefs, or "magical thinking." They may be viewed as eccentric or peculiar, but not psychotic. A person with Schizotypal PD may be overly superstitious, or believe that a random occurrence is part of a design or pattern.

Schizoaffective: A combination of symptoms usually found in Schizophrenia and Affective (mood) disorders. These patients generally exhibit more emotional expression—sadness or joy—than those with Schizophrenia.

Schizophrenia: A major psychiatric disorder, usually having its onset in the teen years or early twenties. Patients often have auditory hallucinations, with visual hallucinations being less common. Delusional thinking, especially paranoid delusions, and disordered or fragmented thoughts are common. These patients have difficulty thinking in abstract terms and tend to be very concrete. They are usually fully oriented to their surroundings, and can answer general questions consistent with their education.

Seizure: See Epilepsy

Self-Mutilation: Deliberately injuring oneself, usually by cutting or burning, to relieve anxiety; or making permanent changes to one's appearance in a manner that is considered unacceptable (in one's culture) or unhealthy. What is acceptable in one culture, such as extensive body piercing or tattoos, may be considered self-mutilation in another.

Tic Disorder: An involuntary muscle spasm or "twitch," usually small, often in the facial area, that repeats with regularity. May increase when the person is tired, under stress, or anxious; and may include cough-like or throat-clearing vocalizations.

Tourette's Syndrome: A tic disorder that may include multiple motor or vocal movements, such as the involuntary repeating or shouting of a word or phrase.

Transsexual: This term refers to individuals who desire to change their physical gender, surgically if possible. Transsexuals will often describe themselves as feeling "trapped in the wrong body," as though they *are* a person of the opposite sex, just born with the wrong genitalia.

Transvestite: "Cross-dressing", or transvestitism, is the desire to dress as a person of the opposite sex. A male may simply wear female undergarments concealed under his conventional clothing; but the cross-dressing can also be complete, with full make-up and hairstyle or wig, giving the actual appearance of the opposite sex. Dressing so relieves anxiety or produces a feeling of pleasure. Dressing in clothing characteristic of the opposite sex may or may not produce erotic sexual pleasure for the individual. Transvestites can be heterosexual by preference and may marry.

Part IV.

Appendices

Appendix A

Serendipity: The Miracle Drugs

1. The History of THORAZINE

The psychiatric benefit of Thorazine (generic chlorpromazine) was discovered serendipitously, in 1952. Dr. Henri Laborit, a Parisian military neurosurgeon and researcher, was experimenting with medications that would enhance the effects of anesthesia so that less could be used, thereby reducing the adverse side effects of anesthesia. He noticed a surprising effect with Thorazine: patients became considerably more relaxed, enabling him to operate with much less anesthetic. He was convinced that it had a useful purpose in psychiatry, but had a hard time convincing the psychiatric establishment of the day, which was skeptical of anything other than shock treatment and psychoanalysis for treatment of severe mental disorders. Smith-Kline pharmaceutical purchased the rights to market chlorpromazine under the trade name of Thorazine as an anti-nausea medication. But when a colleague of Dr. Laborit passed the information along to his brother-in-law, Pierre Deniker, a psychiatrist, he decided to test it on his most hopelessly deranged patients.

> The results were stunning. Patients who had stood in one spot without moving for weeks, patients who had to be restrained because of violent behavior, could now make contact with others and be left without supervision. Another psychiatrist reported, "For the first time we could see that they were sick individuals to whom we could now talk."[11]

---

[11] http://www.pbs.org/wgbh/aso/databank/entries/dh52dr.html (accessed 12/29/2007).

In 1954, Thorazine was approved for use as an anti-psychotic medication in the U. S. Still, it is easy to find negative testimonials on the internet and elsewhere denouncing Thorazine and the anti-psychotic medications that followed. These polemics focus on the sedation and occasional appearance of a reduction in emotions of the patients. Some even refer to it as a "chemical lobotomy." However, as described by one of Dr. Deniker's colleagues at St. Anne Hospital in 1949,

> Strangely, this return to calm was accompanied by a lessening in mental confusion and a re-establishment of normal thought processes. Delirious patients admitted to the department a short time previously, who could not give the day, the month or even the year of their hospitalization, or know where they were or the circumstances that had led to their arrival at the hospital, regained their orientation, remembered the beginning of their illness, and began to discuss their case.[12]

But the most striking evidence of the miraculous benefit of Thorazine is told in numbers: In 1953, when the population of the U.S. was around 160 million, the number of patients in mental hospitals had reached 560,000; by 1975, the U.S. population had *risen by one-third* to 215 million, but the number of patients in mental hospitals had *dropped by two-thirds*, to 193,000. "Although the behavior of schizophrenic patients was once considered to be incompatible with independent functioning in society, the drug enabled thousands to lead lives outside psychiatric institutions."[13]

---

[12] *Ten Years that Changed the Face of Mental Illness*, by Jean Thuillier, Translated by Gordon Hickish. Informa Health Care, 1999.

[13] Rosenbloom, M. Chlorpromazine and the Psychopharmacologic Revolution. *JAMA*. 2002;287:1860-1861.

2. The History of ANTIDEPRESSANTS

Similar to the discovery of Thorazine for schizophrenia, "anti-depressant" medications were serendipitously discovered while working with medication initially prescribed for completely different illnesses. Iproniazid and isoniazid — also developed in the early 1950's — were the first modern medications for treatment of tuberculosis (TB). Patients with TB were isolated in sanitoriums, and when they were treated with these medications, the staff noticed that their mood improved significantly. Unsure whether the mood change was a result of the TB getting better, or a direct result of the medication itself, the doctors began using it on patients who were depressed, but otherwise healthy. The depression did indeed get better, and by 1957, isoniazid and iproniazid were being prescribed for depression. Iproniazid, while somewhat more effective for depression, had some significant toxic effects, and was shortly pulled off the market for use with depression.

Isoniazid continued to be used for decades; however, this class of antidepressant (the monoamine oxidase inhibitors, or MAOI's) fell out of favor due to the many food restrictions that accompanied the prescription. Aged cheeses, smoked meats, red wine, and many other foods could produce a severe headache and dangerous increase in blood pressure when eaten by a patient on MAOI antidepressants.

Imipramine is in a different class, the "tricyclics," referring to its three-ring chemical structure. While being tested in patients with schizophrenia, with no success, it was observed to improve the symptoms of depression, lifting the mood and increasing the energy level. Researchers wondered if imipramine were acting as a stimulant — but administering it to non-depressed patients merely made them fall asleep. "These effects led to the idea that imipramine was selectively reversing the depression, rather than simply producing a general activating effect."[14]

---

[14] *Drugs and the Brain.* ANTIDEPRESSANTS. by Keith A. Trujillo, Ph.D., and Andrea B. Chinn. California State University, 1996.

2. The History of LITHIUM

The Discovery of Lithium[15]

     Lithium is a chemical element with the symbol "Li" and the chemical number 3. It is a soft alkali metal with a silver-white color. According to theory, lithium was one of the very few elements synthesized in the "Big Bang". Because of the method by which elements are built up by fusion in stars, there is a general trend in the cosmos that the lighter elements are more common. Lithium is the lightest metal and the least dense of all the solid (non-gaseous) elements. For unknown reasons, its quantity has vastly decreased such that it is less common than any of the first 20 elements. The reasons for its disappearance, and the processes by which new lithium is created, continue to be active matters of study in astronomy.

     Petalite (lithium aluminum silicate) was discovered in 1800 by the Portuguese scientist José Bonifácio de Andrade e Silva, who discovered the mineral in a Swedish iron mine on the island of Utö. However, it was not until 1817 that Johan August Arfwedson, then a trainee in the laboratory of Jöns Jakob Berzelius, discovered the presence of the element while analyzing petalite ore. The element formed compounds similar to those of sodium and potassium. Berzelius gave it the name "lithos" (from the Greek word meaning "stone"), to reflect its discovery in a mineral, as opposed to sodium and postassium, which had been discovered in plant tissue. The name was later changed to "lithium" which reflected the standard nomenclature of the elements.

Medicinal use of Lithium

     The Greek physician Galen is thought of as the father of modern medicine. He lived a couple of centuries after the birth of Christ. Galen seemed to have had patients who suffered from

---

[15] http://en.wikipedia.org/wiki/Lithium. Accessed March 6, 2009

bipolar disorder, a condition known then as "lunacy" and "mania," where those affected plunge involuntarily and cyclically into states of depression and mania. It appears that Galen prescribed alkaline spring baths for his patients with mania, and, as it turns out, lithium salts are abundant in many spring waters on the earth.[16]

Following the scientific discovery of the actual element in 1817, lithium proved to be very soluble with uric acid (urate). Thus, during the 19th century, lithium was tried as a treatment for a variety of disorders related to urate accumulation, such as kidney stones, gout and uremia. During the late 1940s, evidence accumulated suggesting cardiac and hypertensive patients would benefit from a salt-free diet and lithium chloride seemed an ideal alternative to table salt (sodium chloride). Medical reports appeared in 1949 describing severe poisonings and three deaths connected with lithium chloride, and drug manufacturers voluntarily withdrew all lithium salts from the market.

Just as the dangers of lithium were becoming apparent, an Australian psychiatrist named John Cade began treating patients with mania using lithium. He too was led to this approach from a focus on lithium's solubility with urate. He had injected guinea pigs with lithium urate and found that they became placid, and somewhat tranquilized. Only later did he determine that the calming effect was from lithium, and not urate[17]. With careful attention to dosage and blood concentration, the effectiveness of lithium for patients with bipolar disorder was slowly established. It was approved by the FDA for the treatment of mania in 1970. Speculating about why lithium was not immediately adopted by the psychiatric profession, Cade stated that a discovery "made by an unknown psychiatrist with no research training, working in a small chronic hospital with primitive techniques and negligible equipment, was not likely to command attention."

Lithium has been the treatment of choice for manic-depressive illness since 1970. In addition to treating mania, lithium

---

[16] ASRC Newsletter, Vol. 3, Issue 1, p. 1. June 2004.
[17] Cade JFJ. Lithium salts in the treatment of psychotic excitement. Med J Aust 1949; 2: 349-52.

is also effective in reversing deep depression, the other mood extreme of manic-depressive illness, and in decreasing the frequency of manic and depressive cycles in patients. Manic-depressive illness is now generally referred to as "bipolar disorder"—the term preferred in the psychiatric community.

While there has been a great deal of success in treating manic-depressive patients with lithium and returning them to a normal life, researchers are not exactly sure how it works. It is a non-addictive and non-sedating medication, but blood levels must be carefully monitored. Lithium is also used to treat people who suffer from recurrent depression that may alternate with "normal" moods, without evidence of manic, "hyper" or euphoric phases.

Before lithium was in general use for the treatment of bipolar disorder, as many as one in five patients with this condition committed suicide. Many who suffered from this illness were never able to live normal, productive lives. Lithium therapy now allows many people with bipolar disorder to participate in ordinary everyday life. Sixty-percent or more of bipolar patients respond well to lithium treatment without serious side effects.[18]

Lithium's introduction as the first modern psychopharmacological agent by John Cade in Melbourne, Australia, initiated a revolution in the treatment of manic-depressive patients. Moreover, despite widening clinical use of several plausible alternative psychopharmacological treatments for mania and bipolar depression, lithium remains unrivaled in its level of scientific support for long-term efficacy in manic-depressive disorders. For the long-term prevention of recurrences of major affective episodes in bipolar disorders, it is a truism that maintenance treatment with lithium is effective.[19]

---

[18] Lithium - History Of Use, John Cade, Administration, Precautions. Science Encyclopedia, Volume 4. http://science.jrank.org/pages/3956/Lithium.html. Accessed March 7, 2009.

[19] Baldessarini RJ, Tondo L. Recurrence risk in bipolar manic-depressive disorders after discontinuing lithium maintenance treatment: an overview. Clin Drug Invest 15(4):337-351, 1998.

Appendix B

Internet Links

Al-Anon/Alateen
http://www.al-anon.alateen.org/

American Academy of Psychiatry and the Law
http://www.aapl.org/

American Association of Geriatric Psychiatry
http://www.aagpgpa.org/

American Board of Forensic Psychiatry
http://www.abfp.com/board.html

American Board of Forensic Psychology
http://www.abfp.com/

American Board of Forensic Toxicology
http://www.abft.org/

American Academy of Child and Adolescent Psychiatry
http://www.aacap.org/

American Medical Student Association
http://www.amsa.org/

American Neuropsychiatric Association
http://www.neuropsychiatry.com/ANPA/index.html

American Psychotherapy Association
http://www.americanpsychotherapy.com/

Association of American Medical Colleges
http://www.aamc.org/

National Alliance for the Mentally Ill (NAMI)
http://www.nami.org/

National Institutes of Mental Health(NIMH)
http://www.nimh.nih.gov/publicat/ocd.cfm

Obsessive-Compulsive Foundation
http://www.ocfoundation.org/

Organ Procurement and Transplantation Network
http://www.OPTN.org/

United Network for Organ Sharing
http://www.UNOS.org

Appendix C

Articles and Publications

By Lorraine S. Roth, M. D.
(formerly Lorraine Sharon, M. D.)

Sharon, L.: Countertransference and the Criminal.
  Psychiatric Annals, Vol. 11 (12): 440/49, December 1981

Sharon, L.: Approaching Homosexuality.
  North Carolina Journal of Mental Health, Vol. X, No. 19,
  Winter 1984, P. 17.

Sharon, L.: Benzodiazepines: Guidelines for use in Correctional
  Facilities.
  Psychosomatics, Vol. 25, No. 10, October, 1984

Sharon, L.: Perr Editorial.
  Letters to the Editor. Psychiatric News. Vol. XX, No. 5,
  3/1/85.

Roth, H., Roth, L.: Book Review of Integrated Psychological
  Therapy for Schizophrenic Patients.
  Psychiatric Services, Summer 1996, Volume 47, Number 8.

Roth, L.: Correction to Article on Fibromyalgia.
  Letters to the Editor. Hospital Physician. November 2002.

Roth, L.: The Obesity Epidemic Debate Continues: A 2-Pronged
  Affront.
  Letters to the Editor. Resident & Staff Physician, Vol. 49,
  No. 8, August 2003, p.8.

Roth, L.: Benzodiazepines and Substance Abuse.
Current Psychiatry, Vol. 2, No. 9, Sept.2003, p.3.

Roth, L.: Use, abuse, or misuse? Knowing when to stop benzodiazepines. Pearls, Current Psychiatry Journal. Vol. 3, No. 1. January, 2004. p. 90.

Roth, L.: Acetaminophen Preferable to Ibuprofen for Pretreatment of Electroconvulsive Therapy-Induced Headache. Journal of Clinical Psychiatry 2004;65;5:726.

Roth, L.: Tarvil for TD: Robbing Peter to Pay Paul?
Federal Practitioner, 2004;21(11):48, 53, 56, 62.

Roth, L.: Progress Notes: 10 do's and don'ts (originally "Top 10 Reasons for Writing a Good Progress Note"): Current Psychiatry, Vol. 4, No. 2, Feb. 2005.

Roth, L: The DSM: Simplify, Clarify.
Psychiatry2005, Vol. 4, Issue No. 8.

Roth, L.: "I Feel Safe Here." Discharging the Undischargeable Patient. Federal Practitioner, 2006;23(3): pp. 43-44, 51-54.

Roth, L.: Defuse patient demands and other difficult behaviors (originally "Six Core Conundrums"). Current Psychiatry, Vol. 5, No. 6 / June 2006.

Roth, L.: Clinical Psychopharmacology: Recognizing and Avoiding Common Pitfalls. Psychiatric Times, July, 2007.

Roth, L: DARE to diagnose Borderline Personality Disorder.
Current Psychiatry, Aug 2007. Vol. 6, No. 8. , p. 112.

Roth, L: Be wary when sociopaths turn on the charm. Current Psychiatry, April 2008. Vol. 7, No. 4, p. 55.

Roth, L.: Clinical Psychopharmacology: Recognizing and Avoiding Common Pitfalls. (Update of article published in the July, 2007 issue of Psychiatric Times). Behavioral Health Trends. May 2008. P. 24-29.

Roth, L: Repeat Admissions to Residential Substance Abuse Treatment Programs. Federal Practitioner. May, 2008. Vol. 25, No. 5, pp 32-36.

BOOK REVIEW:
Seeking a cure for health care. A review of *Sick: The Untold Story of America's Health Care Crisis — and the People Who Pay the Price*, by Jonathan Cohn.
Chicago Sun-Times, April 15, 2007.

***

An updated list of publications can be found on the website, www.DearDrRoth.net.

About the Author

Lorraine Sharon Roth, M. D., graduated from medical school at the University of Texas Medical Branch at Galveston; Psychiatric Residency training at the Duke University Medical Center in Durham, North Carolina; and a Fellowship in Forensic Psychiatry at the Federal Correctional Institution at Butner, North Carolina.

~~~~~~~~~

Lorraine is married to Henry J. Roth, Ph. D. They have three children and two grandchildren.

~~~~~~~~~

Henry is a psychologist and special educator who has worked with special-needs children in both therapeutic day school and residential school environments at the Duke University Department of Psychiatry in Durham, North Carolina; the Sonia Shankman Orthogenic School at the University of Chicago; and the Jewish Children and Family Services of Chicago, Illinois. Henry is the author of two books:

Climbing Jacob's Ladder:
Teaching & Counseling Orthodox Students

Tales From Time-Out

Lorraine's *alter ego* is an artist and cartoonist, and she had the pleasure of illustrating her husband's books.

~~~~~~~~~

More information about the Drs. Roth can be found on their website *www.DearDrRoth.net*.

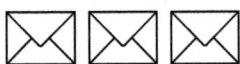

www.ingramcontent.com/pod-product-compliance
Lightning Source LLC
Chambersburg PA
CBHW031955190326
41520CB00007B/258